Finding Your Yoga

Essential Guide to a Healthy Lifestyle
with Yoga and Ayurveda

Urszula Bunting, RYT, CHHC

Finding Your Yoga: Essential Guide to a Healthy Lifestyle with Yoga and Ayurveda

The content for this book is for general instruction only. Each person's physical, emotional, and spiritual condition is unique. The instructions in this book are not intended to replace or interrupt the reader's relationship with a physician or other professional. Please consult your doctor for matters pertaining to your specific health, diet, and exercise.

To contact the author, visit
www.ubwellcafe.com

Internet addresses given in this book were accurate at the time of publication.

Published by UBWell, LLC in the United States of America

Cover Design – Kasia Hypsher
Book Design – Kasia Hypsher
Editing – Regina Stribling
Photography – Kasia Hypsher

Library of Congress Control Number: 2016915001
ISBN: 978-0-9980928-0-5

Dedication

To my sons, Francis and Anthony,
who make my life challenges worth every effort.

CONTENTS

Foreword

Finally, a book that easily describes the ancient practices of yoga, the role it plays in supporting overall health and well being, and the ways that busy individuals can seamlessly incorporate it into their lives. This is great read! This book will leave you feeling inspired and motivated to take charge of your own health in a way that you never have before.

I met Mrs. Urszula Bunting while we were both students at the *Launch Your Dream Book Course* at the Institute of Integrative Nutrition. She is an accomplished yoga instructor and health coach who is passionate about sharing her expertise with the world. As you read this book, you will realize how Urszula's personal experience with yoga has impacted her health in a very positive way. She is teaching from experience, which in my opinion, is one of the best teaching methods. She authored this book as an extension of her love and passion for the practice of yoga, her zest to demystify what it is, and her zeal to help you to *find your yoga.*

As a physician and health coach, with a Masters degree in public health, I understand the importance yoga has on maintain good health. But before reading this book, I also felt that yoga was not for me. I used to think that I was too busy. I thought that I didn't have the right body type for yoga practice to be beneficial to me. I used to think that yoga was just a form of exercise and nothing more. Boy, was I wrong.

After reading this book, I have awakened to the fact that everyone and anyone can and should make the practice of yoga a part of their lives. This book does an excellent job at helping those, who know very little about yoga to understand what it is, and how to slowly add it to their daily lives at their own comfort levels based on their own needs. The chapters in the book give many action steps designed to help even the most inexperienced person start to practice yoga. For me, this book broke down every misconception I had about yoga.

As soon as you begin reading this book, even if you have never tried yoga, you will be inspired and motivated to start immediately where you are at that very point in time. You will learn that you can actually practice yoga anywhere, without necessarily having access to a studio, a mat, or a yoga prop. You can do yoga at home, at work, and while walking, in as little as 10 minutes per day, because as Urszula says, it is your yoga.

As a wife and mother, this book has exemplified ways to introduce healthy yogic lifestyle habits that can be enjoyed by my whole family. I have personally introduced what I call "mini yoga sessions" as part of the bedtime routine for my kids, and I have noticed that they fall asleep faster, have more restful sleep, and wake up more refreshed and ready for each day.

I also enjoy the fact that this book discusses yoga in a holistic fashion by showing how it relates not only to the practices of modern Western medicine, but also to other healing systems of medicine, particularly Ayurveda. Although traditionally thought as an alternative medicine by the Western world, Ayurvedic practices are increasingly being integrated with various Western medicine practices to help patients achieve optimal health and wellness.

This book does a great job at presenting information about the ancient practice of yoga, but in a way that applies to modern times, including specific action steps so you can practice yoga right away. So go ahead, let Urszula help you to find your yoga! She helped me find mine!

Sincerely,

Dr. Rhonda Cambridge-Phillip, MD, MPH, HC
Author of *Bye, Bye Cancer: A Simple Effective Way to Prevent and Heal Cancer*
Brooklyn, NY USA

Introduction

How I Found **My** *Yoga*

I still remember the first yoga class I took at a health club in Connecticut in 1996, when yoga was just becoming popular in the United States. I was young, healthy, flexible, and the type of yoga I chose was a power class. I didn't care about what might have been behind the poses, and why I needed to breathe deeply. All I wanted was to move fast, build a strong and slim body, burn excess energy, and have a good time while doing it. Because I used to dance professionally, getting through the dynamic and challenging poses was relatively easy. I didn't feel the need to further explore the reasons why this kind of exercise was different than others. During that time of my life, yoga was simply a workout.

It wasn't until many years later, after I gave birth to my first child, that I discovered the real meaning of yoga, and its many other benefits. Because my life, my body, and my desires had changed dramatically, I knew that I needed more than just a good workout. I experienced typical challenges as a new mom as well as the challenge that my son was born with severe food allergies (He was allergic to my milk!). I had to learn how to keep my baby safe and healthy while providing the nourishment that he needed to grow. A few months later, I started noticing the effects of being constantly tired, overwhelmed, and worried, in the new reality of motherhood. It was then that I decided to try yoga again. I went to a local yoga studio, put my mat in the corner of the yoga room, and curled up in the first posture, *Balasana*, which means Child's Pose. With my knees bent, hips reaching down toward my heels, and my forehead on the ground–all of a sudden I felt tears coming down my cheeks. First, I noticed how much pain I held in my body, and then I noticed how much I struggled with confusion in my mind. Then, my breath became more relaxed, and my tight body began to release the tension. I stayed in Child's Pose until I was ready to get up, and join the group practice. I didn't even remember what kind of class it was, but it did not matter. It was the day when I found **My** yoga.

Over the years, my practice has changed and developed in support of my needs and my life. Yoga has supported me through the challenges of motherhood, the economy crash in 2008, my husband losing sight in his left eye, and therefore losing his job as an airline pilot, as well as our family's move to Alaska and surviving cold dark winters. Recently my yoga practice has helped me cope with unexpected symptoms of pain, fatigue, brain fog, numerous doctors' visits, and tests that led to a diagnosis of chronic Lyme disease. Yoga has helped me to stay hopeful, remain calm, and see life from a different perspective. It has not only helped me to heal my body, but has allowed me to grow as a person–by finding more gratitude for what I have in my life and more meaning in what I do. Yoga led me to grow professionally–to become a yoga teacher, a health coach, a speaker, and now a writer. Thanks to my yoga practice, my life's difficulties did not take me to a bitter or gloomy place, but rather to a place with more compassion, understanding, and acceptance.

The Purpose of This Book

My main goal for this book is to inspire you to give yoga a try. If you have tried it before, I would like to encourage you to give it another chance. Yoga is a lot more than just doing the poses in a studio or gym. Even though doing it this way can be fun and helpful, I would like to give you the opportunity to start your yoga journey as a way to learn more about yourself in the context of your yoga practice. I would like you to breathe deeply, and become aware of the energy that you generate. To slow down the vortex of your mind in order to think clearly, and thrive in life instead of just barely surviving. Living your life to the fullest potential is possible, and is easier than it sounds. It is a choice. So let's work together. I have chosen to write this book with the hope that you will make a commitment to discover your new path.

In a simple way, I want to show you what I mean by **Your** yoga, and take you on a journey that I hope will lead you way beyond this book into a new discovery of true health and genuine happiness. I want this book to meet you where you are in your life, so look through the pages and see what is there for you. Each chapter is a drop in the ocean. Once you become interested in that drop, I encourage you to dive deeper into an entirely new level of learning and growth.

Why Yoga?

Life is better with yoga! There are many ways to stay sane and healthy in this crazy world of technology, money-driven politics, chronic health conditions, broken relationships, and growing violence. There is something universal and intelligent about yoga that is accessible for everyone. Throughout my experience as a yoga student and a teacher, I have seen many transformations occur because of this incredible 5000-year-old practice.

It's hard not to notice that yoga is very popular these days. Many athletes, movie stars, health experts appear on magazine covers with yoga mats. Many conventional doctors recommend it to their patients for a variety of conditions as an addition to the prescribed treatments. If the politicians in Washington did yoga before making decisions, this might solve many of the problems that Americans are facing now. Yoga is popular simply because it works. It triggers many positive emotions that change the way we perceive the world, which has a significant impact on how we attend to our needs and the needs of others. And it's available for everyone, including regular people like you and me. Whether you're hoping to heal from a chronic condition, prevent diseases, improve your digestion, loose weight, slow down the aging process, manage your stress better, or simply find a community where you feel accepted–yoga offers tools that will support you on your mission.

Writing this book is one of my dreams, and I believe that we can make choices that bring our dreams into reality. My dream for this book is that you find something here that will trigger a change in your life. That it motivates you to make choices for your dreams and desires come true. The tools can be as simple or as complex as you wish, but the results are always priceless. Learning about yourself and about the world around you through the eyes of yoga is a fascinating journey. In our goal-oriented society, it's quite a relief to know that you can enjoy the ride, and not to have to worry about the destination. We all have a responsibility to live our lives to the fullest potential, and to take care of ourselves and the world around us. Yoga makes living our potential: possible, easier, and more fun along the way.

Are you ready? **Let's find Your yoga!**

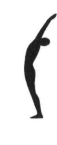

Part One

WHAT IS YOGA? What makes Yoga special?

Chapter 1

Tools of Yoga–The Union of Body, Mind, and Soul

Most yoga instructors love teaching large classes. Mostly because they can sense the positive energy in the room that everyone shares. I also love witnessing people of various ethnic backgrounds, different religions, and opposite political views united together in the pose, the breath, and the experience. It gives me hope for the future of the world–if we can unite on the mat, we can unite off the mat as well.

The word *yoga* comes from Sanskrit, an ancient language from India, the origin of yoga. It means *union* of the body, mind and soul. Very often our minds are troublemakers, and without our intervention, the mind dominates our lives. When the mind gets out of control, it wrecks the body, ignores the soul, and robs us of many great experiences life has to offer. Yoga as a practice offers a collection of tools designed to keep the mind on a leash, bring the awareness to the body, and explore the unlimited potential of the soul. The primary tools and techniques most often used are: breath (pranayama), postures (asana), meditation, chanting (mantra), intention, and visualization.

Breath is a very effective instrument in bringing awareness to the body, and calming the mind. The beauty of this tool is that we all have it built in, but the trick is to learn how to access it and use it consciously. You might think, "what's the big deal, we all breathe." That is true, but unless you are sitting on an island and watching the waves, your breath is probably short, maybe chopped–the exhalations and inhalations are not equal. Stress, illness, and fatigue change the natural patterns of breathing beginning from the time we are born. If you have ever watched a sleeping baby, you might have noticed that her whole body moves as she breaths. The front of her body rises on the inhalation, and sinks on the exhalation. This is the way we should breath all the time, but most often we don't. We have to remind ourselves to let go of gripping the belly, relaxing the ribcage (so the diaphragm can move as we breath), and slowly expanding the chest to make room for fresh air. There are many breathing techniques that are practiced in yoga classes, but my favorite one is observing the breath while inhaling and exhaling through the nose. Interestingly, as soon as we become aware of our breathing pattern, it starts changing, and the breath becomes longer, smoother and deeper. Often our bodies are very tight and the breath does not easily modify old patterns. But there is another tool that comes in handy, and is very effective when practiced on a regular basis. It is the physical part of the yoga practice called *asana*.

Asana is any seated, standing, or reclined posture. Each of the postures has a Sanskrit name and an English translation. For example, *Adho Muka Shvanasana* is translated into *Downward Facing Dog* or an often used "short-cut"–*Down Dog*. The names are not necessary to remember; however, when we continue using Sanskrit words, we honor postures that have been around for thousands of years–they worked then, and they work now. There are hundreds of yoga poses, and each of them can be modified depending on personal needs, preferences and abilities. The six fundamental types of poses that are included in every well-designed practice are: standing poses, forward bends, back bends, balance postures, inversions, and twists.

Standing Poses include: Warriors, Triangle, Chair, and the most fundamental Mountain Pose. Their role is to build strength, flexibility, balance and stamina. They also improve concentration and focus by bringing the body and mind into stillness. Because standing poses are more energizing than seated or reclined postures, they are better to practice in the morning or during the day.

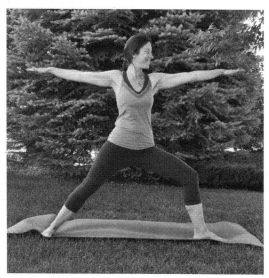

Warrior II Pose

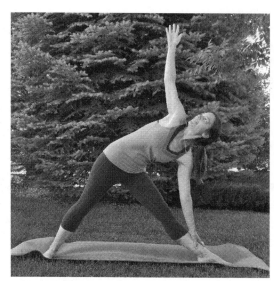

Triangle Pose

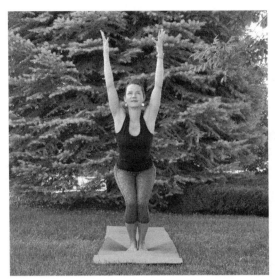

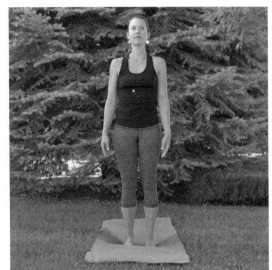

Chair Pose   Mountain Pose

Forward Bending Poses: Child's Pose, Pyramid, or seated Forward Fold. The intention of these poses is to bring more flexibility, especially to the lower back, but also to the upper back, hamstrings, and calves. They are calming to the nervous system when held for a longer time (1-3 minutes) while breathing deeply. Forward bends can be practiced standing, seated, or supine. They can be modified as needed, mainly to keep the lower back safe and healthy.

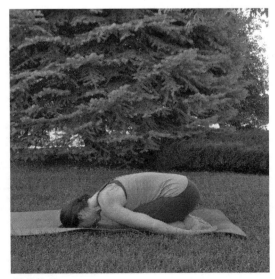

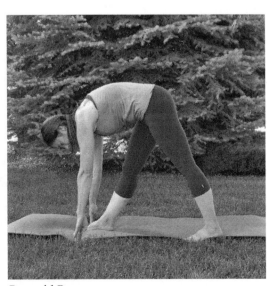

Child's Pose   Pyramid Pose

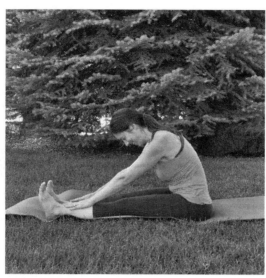

Seated Forward Fold

Back Bending Poses: Cobra, Camel, or Dancer. These are a vital part of a yoga routine. They are also more intense than other postures, and should be practiced only after a good warm up. They are invigorating, uplifting, and heart opening. If done mindfully, they are a great way to keep the spine healthy by stopping or even reversing any damage that might be present in the body from bad posture received from sitting at the computer, driving a car, or a stressful environment.

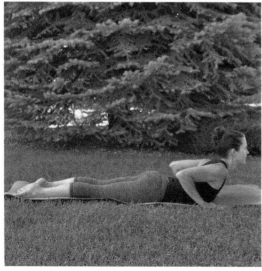

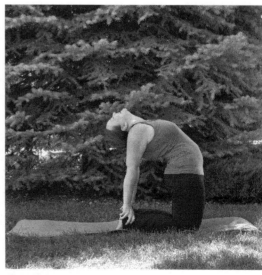

Cobra Pose   Camel Pose

Balance Poses: Tree Pose, Dancer, or Eagle. These poses come in handy for preserving proper balance as we age, and also preventing falls and injuries. They also teach us patience, something that might not come easily, but very useful to master. One of the most popular and less intense balance postures is a Tree Pose–standing on one foot with arms stretched up towards the sky. Others like Dancer or Eagle require more strength and . . . more patience.

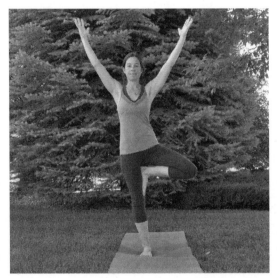

Tree Pose

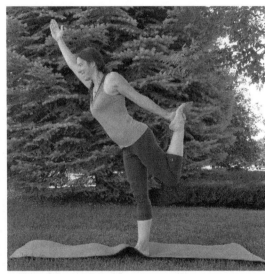

Dancer Pose

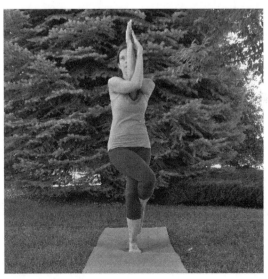

Eagle Pose

Inversions: Down Dog, Bridge, or Legs Up the Wall. These poses are probably the most controversial and misunderstood yoga poses. Most of the time we picture inversions as someone standing on his/her head or hands, but these are advanced inversions that require regular practice, good alignment, and body strength. There are many other inverted poses that can be practiced by anyone, not only seasoned yogis. Anytime the hips are higher than the head–it is an inversion. Poses like Down Dog, Bridge, or Legs Up the Wall (my favorite) are great for anyone to practice. The benefits include: getting more blood flow and oxygen to the brain, improving concentration and memory, stimulating the lymph system, and receiving a different perspective on life simply by seeing the world from being upside-down.

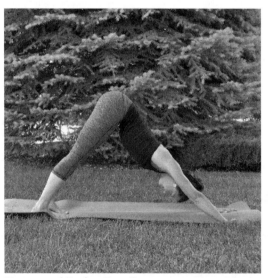

Downward Facing Dog Pose

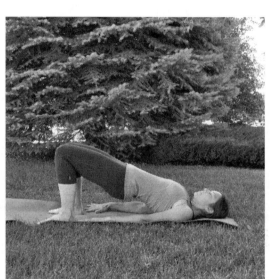

Bridge Pose

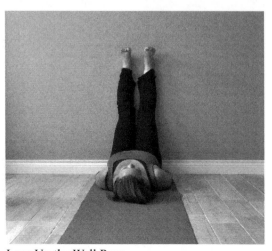

Legs Up the Wall Pose

Twists: These poses are famous for aiding digestion, and easing back pain. Twisted postures are sort of like squeezing a sponge to remove toxins and release tightness that causes backaches. However, I have seen people with back injuries go into twists too fast, or too deep which makes their conditions worse. The most gentle and effective way is to do twists while lying down on the floor, moving slowly and mindfully, focusing on deep and steady breathing. Other examples of twists are: Lord of Fishes Pose, and Revolved Triangle.

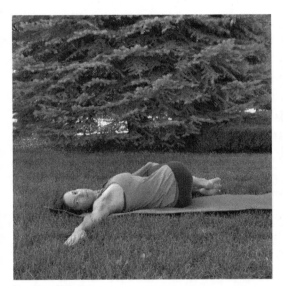

Reclined Twist

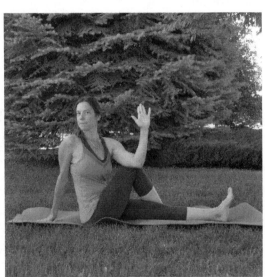

Lord of the Fishes Pose

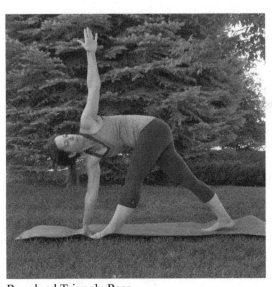

Revolved Triangle Pose

Even though each yoga posture has a focus on a particular area of the body, they all work simultaneously on the whole system. They balance hormones, stimulate digestion, calm the nervous system, improve circulation, promote detoxification, and enhance the respiratory functions. The physical part of the practice is necessary to maintain our bodies to stay in good shape, but for many other reasons besides fitting into tight jeans. The reason is to grow a healthy spirit in a healthy body.

Meditation is when most of the spiritual growth happens–when the mind becomes silent, and inner wisdom surfaces. This is also the time when we heal physically and emotionally, while also discovering who we are by learning about our individual life purpose. Scary? Yes, it can be. We might not like our current situation, but it's what we know. If what we know is sitting in front of the TV for hours, then sitting in silence for five minutes might be very difficult to accomplish at first. It takes time and practice to be ready for a change. Meditation does not have to be torture; it can include walking in the park, literally! Eventually, it is important to progress into a seated meditation, but there are many ways to get there. Finding your favorite way is the first step in the right direction. Walking with awareness, Tai Chi (an ancient Chinese martial art tradition), dancing, asana (meditation in motion), or non-dynamic methods like painting, writing, reading, praying, listening and/or playing music, and singing. These examples of meditation practices help to calm the mind, relax the body, and smooth the breath. The most important point about meditation is to practice it daily, even for a few minutes, to establish new habits and wait for the changes in life to happen painlessly.

Chanting, Intention, and **Visualization** are often, but not always included in every yoga practice. They are excellent tools for people that are looking for a more spiritual type of practice. They add more meaning and assist the practitioner with becoming more grounded and centered. **Intention** is what connects the practice with a person's values and desires, on and off the mat. It is the internal voice coming from the heart that whispers what the true values and desires are. Intention is usually set at the beginning of the practice in order to find this internal voice, and to remain motivated and focused during the practice. Some examples of intentions are: focusing on the breath, staying present, building physical and/or emotional strength, or finding balance on and off the mat. Other more meaningful examples contain elements of gratitude, forgiveness, intuition, love, and trust. Intention is a powerful tool during yoga practice, and it is very helpful when practiced on regular basis. **Chanting** is as simple as saying "Ohm" or as complex as singing or repeating words, sounds, or statements pronounced in Sanskrit from the yogic tradition. However, it can be any word or sentence in any language, from any tradition, that "speaks" to you and helps to focus your mind. **Visualization** is a very effective relaxation practice that uses our imagination to take our mind into a tranquil place to calm the nervous system and relax the body. It is often offered during *Shavasana* (Corpse Pose) that occurs at the end of the practice. Shavasana is the most important part of any yoga practice, and is often the most difficult pose for people to remain in the present moment. During the Corpse Pose, the body rests, but the mind often wanders off. Visualization comes in handy to keep the mind on track for a few more vital moments as a way for the body to absorb and assimilate the benefits of the practice.

Chapter 2

How Did Yoga Begin?

Yoga has a long history and a beautiful philosophy. Every so often we hear that it began 5,000 years ago in India, but there was no written evidence until the second century when Patanjali compiled yoga materials and traditions into a written document. Even Patanjali was a mysterious character, and there is not a lot of information about him. However, we know that he was an Indian sage who brilliantly put together 196 aphorisms and created a text called *Yoga Sutras*, a guidebook, used to this day by yoga followers.

The most well-known and popular part of the *Yoga Sutras* is called "Eight Limbs of Yoga". It describes in a simple and concise way, how to understand the practice of yoga and what to expect in return. It is a road map to a healthier body, calmer mind, and a happier life. In today's culture, we are accustomed to outsourcing so many things, including our health and happiness, to other people and institutions. It is quite an enlightening experience to realize that we may achieve health and happiness on our own. Knowing that we are in the driver's seat is both intimidating and empowering. And yet, following the path that Patanjali gives us, and implementing it in daily routine, transforms the way we face life's challenges.

First Limb of Yoga (Yama) is about ethics and integrity. This limb is broken down into five moral ideals giving us an ethical code, and foundation for our yoga practice. The five moral ideals are: non-violence, truthfulness, non-stealing, continence (self-control in regard to sexual activities), and non-attachment (not being greedy). It reminds us of the simple truth: " treat others they way you want to be treated".

Try this: Choose one day to pay attention to one of the yamas. For example, practice truthfulness and notice if you can catch yourself when you are telling a white lie or making something up in your head that might not be true. Then, consciously lead yourself away from these thoughts or actions.

The second Limb of Yoga (Niyama) is about how to take care of yourself, the importance of self-discipline, and spiritual practice. Similar to the first limb, this one also consists of five principles: cleanliness (inner and outer), contentment (being happy with what you have), austerity (keeping the body in a good condition by paying attention to posture, eating habits, breathing patterns, etc.), studying sacred texts (also self-study and self-examination), as well as letting go of the false impression that you are always in control.

Try this: Choose a Niyama that you would like to work on today. Perhaps cleaning up your desk, or slowing down as you eat, or paying attention to your posture, or being grateful for everything that you have, or letting go of a toxic emotion.

Third Limb (Asana) is about physical postures. The postures are designed to build strength, flexibility, balance, melt away tension, get rid of toxins, and improve the circulation and function of internal organs. Asana is often used as a form of exercise.

Try this: Sit on the floor with your legs crossed in front of you. Inhale and stretch your arms up, exhale and slowly bring them down. Keeping the sitting bones rooted down, extend the arms up, bring the palms together, and slowly bend to one side and the other side. Inhale to lengthen the spine and turn the torso to left as you exhale, come back to the center, and turn to the right with the next out breath. Stretch your legs straight out in front of you, and fold over your legs. Come back up, interlace your hands behind your back (at the base of the spine), and gently lift your chest up as you are bending backward. Release the pose, and take a moment to breathe. Notice how you feel. You can do this entire sequence sitting in a chair or standing.

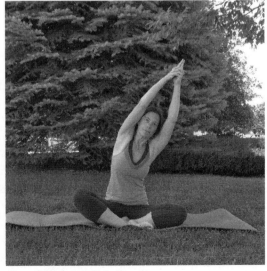

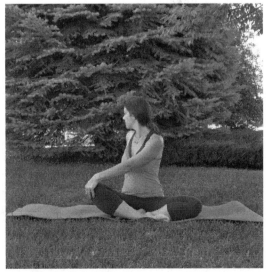

Crossed-legged Side Bend   Crossed-legged Twist

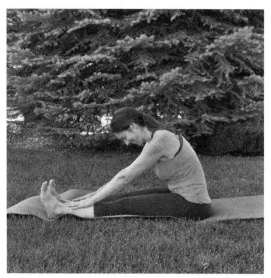

Seated Forward Bend

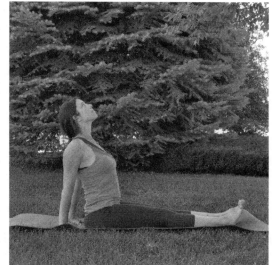

Seated Back Bend

Fourth Limb (Pranayama) is about conscious breathing–a liaison between body, mind and emotions. Breath is an amazing tool that moves the energy called *prana* (life force), relaxes the body, and slows down the mind. The breath works as a guide during the asana practice, and transmits information to the mind such as when to slow down, and when to take a break.

Try this: Lie down on the floor or bed and close your eyes. Place your hands on your lower abdomen, relax your belly, and soften your ribcage and chest. As you inhale, let the breath move down towards the belly, and inflate it like a balloon, then slowly exhale, let the air out and retract the abdomen. Continue several more times, and work on making each breath longer, deeper, and smoother.

Fifth Limb (Pratyahara) is about the importance of tuning inward; to learn how to not be disturbed by outside distractions picked up by the senses. I often ask students to listen to their bodies, breathe and watch the world inside. I find this practice to be very helpful not only during class, but also in a noisy, visually stimulated environment.

Try this: Take a seat and notice the colors, lights, sounds, and scents in the room. Now, close your eyes, relax your face, and feel your breath. Think about the amazing ways the breath and the entire body functions to keep you going no matter your circumstances. After a few moments make an observation about a sound, a color, or anything else that you noticed before you closed your eyes.

Sixth Limb (Dharana) is about the importance of focus. It's not easy to concentrate with many distractions that are constantly bombarding us from all directions. That is why it's important to make the sixth limb a part of our daily practice.

Try this: Take a walk (best done in nature), and try to focus on every step you take.

Seventh Limb (Dhyana) is about being in the present moment, which in simple words describes meditation. Being present requires quite a bit of concentration in dealing with thoughts that usually enter from the past or the future. Seated meditation is what yoga philosophy encourages, but it can be done in many ways, in several positions, and at any time. The best time for meditation is in the morning when your mind is still, not too busy, and can slowly transition from sleep into the day. Just like playing an instrument, meditation requires practice and commitment to see the results.

Try this: Sit down and lengthen your spine. Close your eyes and focus on your breath as it comes in on the inhalation and exits on the exhalation. When your thoughts begin arising, just observe them and let them move away like puffy clouds in the sky. Repeat this exercise every day for a week, preferably at the same time each day. After a week, evaluate the effect of this meditation on your wellbeing. Recommit and do it again for another week, and another week until it becomes a habit.

Eighth Limb (Samadhi) is the last step and the ultimate goal of yoga practice. It is the step where all of the previous limbs come together. The state of harmony between body, mind, and soul united with the universe. It is an experience beyond "me", "I", or "mine" that brings true joy and peace.

Try this: Take a yoga class or do yoga practice at home for 10–15 minutes using poses that you know. Remember to breathe and be mindful of the present moment. At the end of your practice take the last pose, Shavasana, lying down on your back with your legs slightly apart and arms a few inches away from your torso. Close your eyes and breathe naturally. There is nothing else for you to do right now except to surrender for a few precious moments.

Even though Patanjali expresses the importance of developing a spiritual life, it is essential to understand that **yoga is not a religion**. My faith deepened when I started practicing yoga. It did not take me away from what I had already believed and practiced, but instead encouraged me to explore my faith further and become more spiritual. We all have a responsibility to use our body and mind as a contribution to the world. Yoga made my contribution more significant when I started practicing and later teaching.

From my observation, many religions don't emphasize the importance of taking care of ourselves to be better at serving others. According to yoga philosophy, "the body is a temple". No matter what kind of temple it is, it still needs to be maintained in order to grow, and be shared with others. The *Eight Limbs of Yoga* are universal truths that can fit into many cultures and beliefs. The best thing about yoga is that it encourages you to listen to your body and listen to your heart. If chanting in Sanskrit, bowing at the end of the yoga class, or seating for meditation does not seem right for you, simply don't do it. Find your way to practice yoga, and remain loyal to your tradition and faith.

Chapter 3

One Yoga, Many Styles

The first time people in America heard about yoga was over one hundred years ago when Swami Vivekananda, an Indian monk, came to the World's Columbian Exposition in Chicago in 1893 to represent India and Hinduism *(McCall, 10)*. Eighty years later the first yoga studio opened in New York City. Now, yoga is a multi-billion dollar industry selling clothing, accessories, mats, blankets, blocks, towels, and more. Thousands of people have become instructors around the country; opening studios in almost every town, and offering classes in the YMCA, gyms, hospitals, as well as recreation, community, and senior centers. It's estimated that in the United States, over twenty million people are doing yoga. Yes, we live in a country that can turn anything popular into a money making machine. But that's what keeps the economy going, and makes the country prosperous. In terms of yoga practice, it's best not to get caught up in popular brands nor allow the industry to make choices for you. If wearing brand-name clothing during yoga classes makes you feel more motivated, go for it, but don't let this be the determining factor. Lululemon (a brand that makes flattering yoga pants) will not increase the benefits of your practice, simply make it a little more expensive.

Today, we have many modern styles of yoga that serve just about everyone: from athletes to people with compromised movement, from babies to older adults, from those who are looking for a good workout to others that want to transform their lives. Depending on your desires and abilities, you can find classes that are fast or slow, healing and therapeutic, powerful or gentle, prenatal and postnatal, taught in a heated room, or practiced in the park. Styles like Hatha, Vinyasa, Ashtanga, Bikram, Iyengar, Yin, and Anusara have names that are less informative about the style, so it's a good idea to find out about the classes before attending one. In this chapter, you will have a chance to learn about each style including what each style has to offer, and how each style is different from another. Based on this information you will be able to choose the style that seems right for you. Then you will be able to locate a teacher you enjoy that provides classes in a space where you can relax with a group of people that shares similar energy. After that, the practice is up to you. No matter what the style is or what the instructor says, it's your practice. Your body and your breath are your best guides and teachers, so always listen to them.

Finding the style and the practice that is right for you might take a few attempts, so don't become discouraged if it doesn't happen right away. You will know when you find what works for you. It will feel like coming back home after a long and tiring trip. It takes a couple of months to learn the postures, and to understand how your body responds to them. It takes even longer to change old habits, and invite in new ones. It takes a lifetime to learn who you are, and become comfortable with what you find out. Just like starting any new journey, yoga also requires some patience and persistence, but it does get easier and more pleasurable as you become more familiar with the postures and techniques. When you start noticing the benefits, you will never want to quit.

Hatha Yoga is one of the six original branches of yoga and is the foundation for most of the modern styles. Hatha also means balance (*Ha* translates as sun and *Tha* translates as moon). Almost any style of yoga available today can be interpreted as a customized Hatha style *(Stephens, 17)*. Classes that are advertised as Hatha Yoga are usually gentle, and postures are held for a few breaths or longer. Hatha style is a great choice for beginners, and anyone who likes to move at a slower pace. Hatha Yoga classes can vary a great deal depending upon the instructor, and how she or he interprets this style of yoga.

Vinyasa, also called **Vinyasa Flow**, is the most popular style in the West, in particular among the younger generation. Vinyasa means moving with the breath. The sequence is usually designed in a way that the body moves from posture to posture without stopping in between, which often resembles dancing. The pace is faster, stimulating, and energizing. A Vinyasa class is fun to do in the morning or during the day for a quick "pick me up".

Ashtanga is a form of Vinyasa, or rather the Vinyasa style has its roots in Ashtanga. A traditional Ashtanga class is very specific. The postures are always the same, practiced in the same order while every movement is linked with the breath. You can find many studios around the country that offer this style, but only some of them follow the original concept where each student moves through the sequence of postures on his/her own, and the teacher is there to give individual instructions to the students. In most Ashtanga classes, the instructor leads the whole practice at the same pace with instructions that apply to the whole group of practitioners. Traditional Ashtanga is based on the Yoga Sutras, and is a very focused and intense practice.

Power Yoga is a more vigorous and fitness oriented form of Vinyasa. It also has roots in the Ashtanga style, but each class does not necessarily have the same sequence of postures. This style is often offered in gyms and fitness clubs, and is very popular among athletes. People attracted to this style often have three main goals: to build strength, flexibility, and endurance.

Hot Yoga represents any style practiced in a heated (95-105 degrees) room. Most of the time the style is a Vinyasa or Bikram yoga. **Bikram** style yoga was invented by Choudhury Bikram, an instructor who came to the United States from India. He opened his first studios in Hollywood, CA in 1970s and 1980s. Since then, this style has gained a lot of popularity around the country and other parts of the world through the design of a 90-minute practice consisting of 26 postures performed in a heated room (105 degrees and 40 percent humidity). The postures and the sequence are always the same performed twice. Hot yoga feels good because the heat helps to stretch muscles, loosen up joints, and detoxify the body through sweating. However, this style is not for everyone. People that have health concerns like high blood pressure, heart disease, or chronic inflammation should try a different style, or at least, talk to a health care professional before beginning a Hot Yoga class. It's also important to be very mindful while practicing at a high temperature–not to overstretch, which can lead to injuries.

Iyengar yoga is named after its founder B.K.S Iyengar, who was born at the beginning of the 20th century in India. During his childhood and adolescence, B.K.S Iyengar experienced poor health and difficult life circumstances. In search of wellbeing, he started his yoga practice by experimenting with Hatha yoga and eventually became a very accomplished teacher. Iyengar Yoga is a style that is very precise, and based on alignment of body parts to protect them and to ensure the energy flow. The use of various props (blocks, blankets, belts, chairs) and posture modifications make this form of yoga not only accessible, but also safe and effective for anyone who might have limitations *(Stephens, 34-35)*. Certification in Iyengar yoga requires many years of rigorous training, which means that the certified instructors are very knowledgeable and experienced with accommodating students' individual needs.

Anusara is a relatively new form of Hatha Yoga invented by John Friend in 1997, who previously was a student of the Iyengar style. The English translation of Anusara is "following your heart" or "going with the flow". The Anusara community has a very positive approach, and is open to students of all levels. With the use of props, it accommodates practitioners' needs and allows the students to "explore" their potentials while practicing the postures, following the breath, and connecting body, mind, and soul in a positive and non-rigid way.

Kundalini Yoga is an ancient practice where the emphasis is on the breath, chanting and meditation in search of spiritual awakening. The sequences of postures are called kriyas, and many of them are quite different from sequences typically used in other styles. In some kriyas, poses are held for several minutes while also breathing and repeating a mantra. However, most of the time the sequence is fast with repetitive movements, vigorous breathing, and silent repetition of a mantra. This style is one of the most spiritual. It can also be very intense physically and emotionally. If you walk into a room where Kundalini yoga is being practiced, you will know right away because the teachers (and some students) wear white clothes, white turbans, and sometimes use white sheep's skin instead of yoga mats on the floor.

Yin Yoga is a much more passive practice consisting of a fewer number of poses that are held for at least five minutes, and most of them are done while lying down on the floor. Yin yoga targets deep connective tissue and fascia in the body, and lubricates joints and ligaments. Compared with other styles where big muscles are being stretched and strengthened, Yin yoga helps to bring more flexibility, especially into the hips, sacrum and spine. The poses also work on emotional issues that contribute to tightness in those areas.

Restorative Yoga is truly for everyone. It brings balance to the body and mind, something that we are missing in life these days. People who are very active need to slow down and "catch their breaths", while people that are not active enough need to find motivation to start moving forward. Restorative practice helps address many issues including: stress, fatigue, recovery from illness, pain, chronic conditions, or simply getting a break from life challenges. The main purpose of Restorative yoga is to trigger the natural healing process. I discovered Restorative yoga when I learned that I had chronic Lyme disease. This style of yoga became my essential medicine for restoring my health and wellbeing. While I struggled with pain and fatigue, sometimes not able to move vigorously, I practiced poses for my body to rest and restore. By gently stretching, my mind remained calm, and all of the systems of my body returned to balance. It worked for me, and I have seen it work for many other people. During a Restorative class, you lay down on the floor propped with blankets, blocks, bolsters, and pillows–to bring maximum comfort to your body with minimum effort. Being comfortable in this way, allows the parasympathetic nervous system to become activated so that your body can fully relax. Doesn't that sound good?

Prenatal Yoga is specifically designed to keep pregnant women safe during asana and breathing practices. Practicing yoga during pregnancy has many benefits for the mom and the baby including: preparing for childbirth, staying fit, sleeping better, reducing stress and anxiety, and decreasing low back pain and nausea. There are some poses (deep twists, beckbends, forward folds, and a few breathing techniques) that are not appropriate during pregnancy, therefore it's always a good idea to take a class with a teacher that is trained in prenatal yoga.

Yoga Therapy is a new healing/therapeutic concept that is currently being considered by Western medicine as an addition to traditional treatments. Yoga, in general, is a therapeutic discipline, but yoga therapy is designed to address specific health concerns. Practitioners work individually or in small group settings to receive a lot of individual attention. Yoga therapists are usually yoga instructors whom have additional training in yoga philosophy, anatomy, and physiology. They have a more thorough understanding of postures and modifications as well as Ayurvedic and other alternative approaches to healing.

There are many more styles of yoga "on the market", and I am sure there will be even more as yoga's popularity continues to grow, and I believe it will. No matter which style you choose, remember that there is only one yoga–**Your Yoga**. What matters is that you find what works for you and ideally practice it every day. Even if it's only for a few minutes, even if all you can do is take a few conscious breaths, even if it's checking in with your heart and soul–it is your journey, and it begins with taking small steps. When you become serious about yoga, look for an instructor that is right for you rather than a specific style of yoga. Most of the yoga instructors are very dedicated, disciplined, and know their stuff. Yoga instructors attend more continuing education seminars, self-care programs, and professional growth training than any other professional I know. Begin by talking to the instructor, taking the class, and listening to the feedback your heart gives you.

Chapter 4

Yoga is Not Just For Women!

Whether you are a man or a woman, a child or an adult, single or married, an accomplished athlete, or someone with compromised fitness ability, you like the rest of us, experience life challenges that are often hard to avoid. When your world starts falling apart, it is fundamental to have your faith, community, physical wellbeing, and sense of emotional strength to get you through the rough times, and move on with your life without scars. Regular yoga practice has a way to develop each of these elements, helping you to navigate through the stormy periods, and bring more enjoyment to happy moments. Yoga is a gift that I would love everyone to discover, and unwrap it—one layer at the time.

For Men

Despite its popularity and proven benefits to both genders, modern yoga is dominated by women. Only about 20 percent of yoga students are men, which is fascinating because the first yogis were men! Yoga was originally developed, studied, and practiced by monks in ancient India. Many modern styles of yoga were invented and taught by men. So why don't men attend yoga classes as much as women do? Perhaps because yoga studios are filled with women, it gives the wrong impression that yoga has a feminine profile, and somehow practicing yoga will negatively effect the masculine side of men. Also, men often think they are not flexible, and yoga is only for people that are. For some men, yoga is too passive and does not look like a good workout, so they would rather lift weights, use gym equipment, or get involved in sports.

Over the years of teaching yoga, I have had many men in my classes. I truly enjoy working with them. I have worked with athletes, soldiers, firefighters, police officers, pilots, doctors, businessmen, teachers, and college students. Their physical and emotional strength proved to me that yoga does not make a man less of a man, and it's not just for people that are already flexible. No matter the level of personal strength and flexibility, yoga builds more of it. Yoga helps with self-esteem and confidence. It contributes to men being more masculine, and very attractive! Typically women love having men in the yoga room. In the end, yoga is a union, and it's all about balance. Once men find the yoga style that is right for them, the teacher that speaks their language, and the environment that feels comfortable, they become very committed, focused and centered.

Try this: If you have never tried yoga before, find a class that is for beginners and attend it at least once a week for two months. During that time try not to analyze it too much, just go with the flow. After two months, decide if the class is for you, and either continue, find another class, or implement what you have learned in your exercise routine.

For Athletes (Men and Women)

Yoga is a great addition to many sports like: skiing, running, golf, bicycling, weight lifting, and more. I have taught yoga in a country club where many of my students were golfers. Most of them reported to me that their golf scores were much better since they started attending yoga classes. This is what one golfer had to say:

"Yoga helps me with flexibility which is important because the more flexible I am, the better my golf swing is. I play in national golf tournaments and the more flexible I am, the more I can compete against guys half my age."

Yoga works on many levels, but for anyone that is involved in sports, yoga is an excellent way to evenly strengthen the entire body, stretch muscles, lubricate joints, and stretch tendons. All of which helps athletes avoid injuries, and receive better results especially in competitive sports. Including a slower pace yoga practice (Restorative or Yin) to an athlete's exercise routine, helps calm the nervous system, and provide the body with the quality rest needed among high achievers.

Try this: Next time when you're ready to do your exercise routine or a sports activity, instead of rushing straight to it, slow down, take several deep breaths, and relax any muscles that might be tense. For a moment, allow yourself to tune inside: observe your breath, your heartbeat, and your pulses rather than think about what you are going to do next. Feel the ground under your feet, stretch your arms up above your head, lengthen your spine, and lift your chest up towards the sky. Breathe and observe. Now you're ready for your workout, game, or tournament.

For Couples

I have always enjoyed seeing couples taking yoga classes together. What a wonderful way to spend more time with one another while getting healthier! In my opinion, yoga helps couples better understand each other, be more accepting and forgiving, and support each other on and off the mat. All of these qualities make the relationship stronger, and persevere through difficulties. There is no secret that the divorce rate is very high in the United States and other western countries. Very often couples simply grow apart, and realize that they have very little in common. Practicing yoga together might be the thing that keeps them together, and helps them fall in love with each other over and over again. No guarantees, but worth trying.

There are poses that are designed for two people to do together. Some instructors incorporate these poses in their classes. Doing yoga as a couple is simply about being on the mat next to one another, hearing his or her breath, feeling the energy, letting go of the differences and experiencing the connection that contributes to long lasting love and commitment.

Try this: Visit a yoga studio in your area and talk to the instructor to find out what class he or she would recommend for you and your life partner. Make it a date. Take a class together, and after the class spend more time with each other doing something that you both enjoy.

For Children
Today, kids are stressed out more than ever before. Have you ever watched a child playing video games? Their breathing becomes shallow, their bodies become tight, and their faces become frozen from tension. With numerous academic tests, and often not enough play time, kids have difficulties in developing a healthy view of life from the fast paced world around them. The tools used in yoga (breathing, visualization, and gentle movement in a safe and noncompetitive environment) can make a huge difference in how a child handles his/her emotions and deals with stress. Yoga helps children develop interpersonal skills, which are rapidly declining in the age of texting, emailing, Facebook, and other technological social interactions. Yoga also creates a nonjudgmental environment that helps kids to learn to respect others and their choices. As a form of art, yoga gives children the opportunity to acquire creativity, something that is essential for surviving and thriving later in life. Yoga postures help boost confidence, build self-awareness, improve motor skills and calm the nervous system. Therefore, yoga can also be a very useful tool as part of a therapy plan for children with ADHD/ADD, Autism, and other learning, behavioral, and emotional disorders.

Kids' Yoga classes are often offered for participants of a variety of ages, and support specific attention spans, interests, and a range of possibilities. Children that are in a well-designed and fun class truly thrive; the benefits are quickly noticeable. Working with children is very rewarding because the results are much faster since children have few boundaries and very little emotional luggage that can take years to unload. Yoga for Kids is offered at yoga studios, recreation centers, and after school programs. The most important aspect is to be sure that the instructor has experience with teaching yoga to children, and that he or she has received additional training in this particular type of yoga. Most of the time, yoga practice for children includes: postures, breath work, guided imagery, and sometimes meditation. However, it's a lot more playful and fun than the adult version. Just a few simple poses practiced every day (Down Dog, Tree, Child's Pose) can significantly improve a child's life and the life of the whole family.

Try this: After a busy day, practice a short yoga sequence with your children. Invite your child/children to take a seat in a crossed legged position (criss-cross apple sauce). Close your eyes, and take a few conscious breaths through the nose. Feel the breath as it comes in on the inhalation and exits on the exhalation. Bring your legs into a wide straddle and fold forward keeping your spine long and straight with your hands on the floor. Hold the position for a few breaths and come back up. Come onto all fours to continue with Cat and Cow postures: inhale, lift the sitting bones up, arch the spine, and lift the head up; exhale, curl the tailbone, round the spine, and relax the head down. Repeat several times. Walk your hands a few inches forward, press your palms to the floor and lift your hips up into Down Dog. Slowly straighten the knees and bring the heels closer to the floor. Hold for several deep breaths. Lie down on your back in Shavasana with your arms a few inches away from the torso and legs a few inches apart. Let the breath become naturally deep and smooth. Observe your breath, and encourage your child to do the same for a few precious minutes.

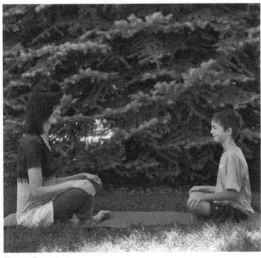

Easy Pose

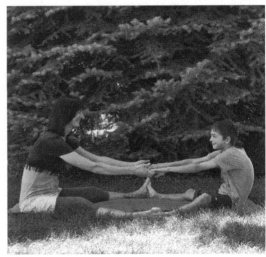

Wide Straddle Forward Bend

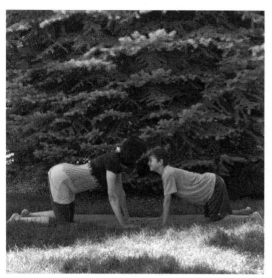

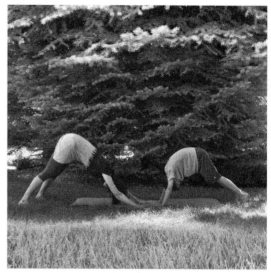

Cat and Cow Postures   Downward Facing Dog Pose

For Anybody and Everybody!
I might be biased, but people that practice yoga are not only healthier, but are happier, too. Here is something I heard from one of my students:

"I have never seen a grumpy person leave a yoga room".

No matter your age, your gender, your profession, or level of fitness, you can practice yoga at your comfort level. You deserve to be **healthy** and **happy**!

Part Two

YOGA AND AYURVEDA: The Perfect Couple

Chapter 5

Why Ayurveda?

Yoga is a form of exercise, and also a way of life. Once you learn about postures, conscious breathing, and slowing down the vortex of the mind, most likely you will become curious about other lifestyle changes that can support your wellbeing. When you start noticing the benefits of yoga, you may realize that life doesn't have to be a constant struggle. You may want to explore other changes you can easily implement in your everyday life such as: eating habits, sleeping patterns, responding to stress, and connecting to nature. Many of the lifestyle changes can be found in the wisdom of an ancient healing tradition called Ayurveda.

Ayurveda is a combination of two Sanskrit words *Ayu* and *Veda*. When put together, it means "science of life" *(Yarema, 20)*. It is holistic medicine from India that has been healing people for thousands of years. Even though it has a very different approach to western medicine, it is similar to other traditional healing systems such as traditional Chinese medicine. The basic principals of Ayurveda are: the focus on prevention, importance of proper digestion, adjusting the lifestyle according to one's constitution, living in tune with nature (eating seasonal foods), getting enough rest, and taking it easy. There is a lot of wisdom in Ayurveda, but mainly a great deal of common sense. It is not uncommon to be confused about how to live a healthy life including: what to eat, how much to exercise, and which health practitioner to follow. One main reason people may have difficulty understanding this ancient science is based on the way we, in the modern world, live our lives that simply does not make sense. Examples of Western habits that don't make sense are: putting artificial food in our bodies, eating raw and cold salads in the winter, eating grilled and greasy meat in the summer, staying up late at night when our biological clock is telling us to go to sleep, not exercising at all or working out too much, and going to work or school while we are sick. These kinds of lifestyle habits are not sustainable in the long run.

Ayurveda recognizes that our bodies are constantly looking for balance, and we can stay in balance if we maintain healthy habits on a regular basis. We have a built-in healing system that simply needs to be activated and maintained. However, health is not effortless, and it takes more than just swallowing pills for the rest of our lives. Ayurvedic lifestyle choices require time and determination. These choices are the difference between thriving and barely surviving. Is it worth it? Absolutely!

My experience with Ayurveda started over a decade ago. I knew a little bit about it from practicing yoga, but not enough to implement it into my lifestyle. At that time, I was desperately looking for help for my three-year-old son who, besides having severe allergies, was getting frequent colds that usually turned into croupy coughs. I was terrified about his health after a conversation I had with another parent, whose slightly older children had similar health issues. His kids were on steroids from September to May each year. Instinctively, I knew that there had to be a different, gentler approach.

To this day, I am grateful that I found a physician who was also an Ayurvedic practitioner. She was my first teacher and motivator. After she had identified my son's constitution and imbalances, she prescribed gentle herbs, healing foods and lifestyle changes. I started using the information I learned from her not only for my son, but for the entire family. Slowly, my son was doing better, and I felt stronger and more at peace. Did Ayurveda fix all of my son's problems? It did not, but it made a huge difference in his health and development without putting him at risk.

There have been many situations where I experienced the healing power of Ayurveda, but one in particular was remarkable. My husband, who was a commercial pilot for over 20 years, had a hemorrhage in his left eye, and lost sight during one of his flights. It was a scary time. I had just given birth to my second child, the economy crashed, and my husband no longer had the job that supported our livelihood. He was evaluated by the best ophthalmologists and surgeons, but they had no answers for him about why this had happened, and whether he was ever going to see and fly again. Even though my husband believed in Western, science-based medicine, in desperation he decided to try something non-conventional. He had already known about the healing power of Ayurveda from the experience with our son, so he was willing to give it a try. He came back from his first visit with our Ayurvedic doctor with a perplexed look on his face and a diagnosis of "too much pitta (heat) in the eye". With no other options and my encouragement, he chose to try the Ayurvedic approach. The healing process was long and slow, but six years later he was flying big jets again!

Yoga and Ayurveda makes a perfect couple. Each of them can exist separately, but they are much better together. They complement each other and work together towards the same goal–true health and real happiness. Both yoga and Ayurveda have a common understanding of how the human body works, what health means, and what role the mind plays in health and wellbeing. Just like yoga, Ayurveda is gaining a lot of popularity in recent years, and it is becoming known as a preventative and holistic healing system. If you become fascinated with an Ayurvedic approach to life and decide to pursue it beyond this book (I hope you will!) there are many books, cookbooks, practitioners, schools, and institutes you can pursue (see Resources in the back of this book). Many yoga instructors are familiar with Ayurveda, and they are an excellent resource on how to find a practitioner in your area.

Chapter 6

Finding Your Constitution

One of the best things about Ayurveda is that it recognizes every human being's unique constitution. Constitution (also called body type or *dosha*) is like a blueprint that we arrive with at birth, and makes us who we are physically and emotionally, as well as how we respond to the environment around us. Our constitution is responsible for our strengths and weaknesses; how we process the information given by life experiences. There are three basic constitutional types in Ayurveda: Vata, Pitta, and Kapha. It's good to know your dosha, and to become aware of whether your lifestyle is truly supporting you or creating imbalances that lead to health problems.

The basic test below will take only a minute, but it will give you a general idea as to who you are physically, emotionally, and mentally from an Ayurvedic perspective. A more accurate assessment can be done by an experienced Ayurvedic practitioner who can establish your constitution using a more comprehensive evaluation including a pulse reading test. Below is a list of terms; circle the ones that describe you the most.

	VATA	**PITTA**	**KAPHA**
Body size	thin	medium	large
Weight	low	medium	rather heavy
Nose	uneven shape	long and pointed	short and rounded
Eyes	small	sharp and bright	big and soft
Skin	dry and thin	smooth and warm	thick and oily
Hair	dry and brittle	straight and fine	thick and oily
Nails	dry and rough	sharp and flexible	thick and smooth
Joints	cracking	flexible	large and lubricated
Digestion	irregular, gassy	strong, steady	slow, with mucus
Elimination	constipation	loose	sluggish
Sleep	light and broken up	moderate and sound	deep and long
Emotions	anxiety, worry	anger, temperamental	calm, attached
Temperament	enthusiastic	purposeful	easy going
Speech	fast, unclear	sharp, effective	slow, monotonous
Intellect	quick but unclear	accurate	slow but exact
Totals			

After you finish, count the answers in each column, and write the number of answers under each column. The highest number of answers indicates your constitution. For example: if under the Vata column you have number 6, under Pitta column number 9, and Kapha column number 3, then you are most likely Pitta type.

In Nature, there exist five elements: space, air, fire, water, and earth. These are the foundation to any material existence, including us. Every one of us has all five elements, but at a different ratios, which means that usually there are two elements that dominate, and these determine the constitution. It happens sometimes that a person has more than two elements that dominate his or her constitution, and this means that the dosha is dual (e.g. Vata-Pitta) or even tri (Vata-Pitta-Kapha). This is one example that demonstrates how Ayurveda is, just like life (remember Ayurveda means "life science"), it's not black and white. The answers are neither always straight nor easy, but that's what makes Ayurveda fascinating and worth exploring.

If you are a Vata type:
You and I might have a lot in common. I am the most typical Vata type I know. The elements of Vata are Space and Air, which means that I am constantly on the move. I have a lot of energy, and I love change, but if I don't slow down when necessary, I get easily depleted. When I am depleted, I become restless. By being restless, I become ungrounded which causes me to become: anxious, worried, constipated, bloated, along with challenges in sleeping soundly. The qualities of Vata are: dry, light, cold, and mobile. To keep myself balanced, I need to apply the opposites of Vata qualities such as: warm climates (I love Hawaii!), warm and oily foods (creamy tasting soups), slow movement, and associate with people that are calm and grounded. When I am balanced, I can be very creative, social, communicative and charismatic. When my Vata gets out of control, then, well . . . you don't want to be around me. Vata means "the wind" and I admit that sometimes I feel like a hurricane, but with the tools that Ayurveda offers I know how to slow down and turn into a breeze. Because the Vata type does not have a strong digestion, Vata people experience a low digestive fire which means they have to pay attention to what they eat, how the food is prepared, and when they have their meals.

This is what I do to keep my Vata happy:

* *Get up early, take a 20-minute walking mediation, and then do 10 minutes of yoga or Tai Chi.*
* *Use the dry brush technique and oil massage before the shower.*
* *Eat meals at regular times in a relaxed atmosphere (I have, to be honest here: it does not always happen, but I keep trying).*

- *Limit cold drinks and raw, cold, and dry foods.*
- *Use lots of olive oil, ghee, and grass-fed butter.*
- *Use warming herbs and spices (turmeric, ginger, cumin, fennel, cardamom, coriander).*
- *Go to bed early–read and pray before falling asleep.*
- *Take a bath once or twice a week with Epsom salt and lavender oil.*
- *Take a gentle or restorative yoga class once or twice a week.*
- *Get a massage at least once a month.*
- *Go to the beach for vacation and walk barefoot on the warm sand (Can't wait!).*

If you are a Pitta type:
Well, you might be a lot like my husband. The elements of Pitta are Fire and Water. The qualities are: oily, sharp, hot, light, liquid and acidic. The Pitta type has a sharp intellect, confidence, sense of humor, strong sense of leadership, incredible determination and courage. However, when out of balance the joyful Pitta turns into an angry fire. The popular saying for Pitta types "Imbalanced Pitta people don't go to hell; they create it" describes this type pretty accurately. Because of the presence of the fire element, the Pitta type has a tendency toward inflammation, acid reflux, hot flashes, canker sores, diarrhea, ulcers, and infections. Anything that is cooling and calming will keep Pitta to become in balance. Pitta has a very strong digestion and can digest almost anything. Before I had learned about doshas, I always wondered why my husband was able to enjoy a big heavy meal and feel good afterwards while I usually had to choose much healthier foods that also came with indigestion at times. Now I know that the answer is a lot more than, "Men are from Mars and Women are from Venus." It's Vata versus Pitta!

This is what people can do to keep their Pitta happy:

- *Meditate daily.*
- *Spend more time in nature: walking, swimming, watching the sunrise or sunset, observing birds, animals, and plants.*
- *Listen to soothing and relaxing music.*
- *Laugh and smile more.*
- *Do a self-massage with cooling oil (coconut) and then take a cool shower.*
- *Make daily journal entries.*
- *Engage in calming physical activities such as Tai Chi, Yoga, walking, or swimming.*
- *Limit refined sugar, alcohol, and caffeine.*
- *Choose healthy cooling foods like salads, fruit, and herbs (mint, Aloe Vera, rose*

water).
- *Drink plenty of water.*

If you are a Kapha type:
No one in my family is a typical Kapha, but I have a lot of friends and students that are Kapha types. I love Kapha people because they are very grounding, and balancing for both Vata and Pitta personalities. These people are the warm, gentle, and loving Teddy Bears that you want to hug so you can melt your tension in their arms. The elements of Kapha are Water and Earth. The qualities are: moist, cold, heavy, soft, and sticky. Typically the Kapha types are the healthiest, and the most resilient among all three doshas. They have a heavier stronger physical structure, and are mentally more peaceful than other types. However, if out of balance, Kapha becomes the famous couch potato. Health problems that Kapha types can encounter are: obesity, diabetes, asthma, sinus congestion, lethargy, and depression.

This is what a Kapha type people can do to stay healthy and happy:

- *Go to bed early and rise early.*
- *Adjust their lifestyles according to seasonal changes in nature (especially during the damp spring that creates more mucus and imbalances for Kapha).*
- *Use a dry sauna.*
- *Spend time with interesting and simulating personalities (balanced Vata and Pitta types).*
- *Engage in physical activities that are energizing and stimulating: Vinyasa Yoga, hiking, biking, jogging, swimming, playing sports, dancing, etcetera.*
- *Eat less in general, but especially less of sugary and greasy foods.*
- *Avoid snacking, eating after dinner, and between meals.*
- *Include lots of veggies, legumes, hot and spicy drinks such as ginger or chai tea.*

If you are a Dual-Doshic type such as Vata-Pitta:
The best way to keep yourself healthy and happy throughout the year is to pay more attention to the Vata qualities during the fall and winter months, when Vata is most vulnerable, then adjust diet and lifestyle in the spring and summer months when Pitta has more fire, and a tendency to become out of balance. Similarly, Pitta-Kapha and Vata-Kapha need to adjust with the seasons and nourish the doshas that are most susceptible at that time of the year.

Not that long ago, I listened to my sons arguing in the car. After my nine-year-old could not find any other ways to argue with his older brother, he said: "Because you are just a Pitta, Pitta, Pitta!!!" On a more serious note, having a basic understanding of the different constitutions is helpful, not only for your sake, but it also helps with cultivating more compassion and less judgment with other people. So next time when you see someone anxious, frazzled, and about to lose control over her emotions in the middle of cold and windy winter day–give her a cup of warm soup and a big hug. Or if you look at an overweight individual with criticism, consider giving him some encouragement and motivation to get his Kapha moving. Instead of judging someone as being an angry person, you might look at him or her with compassion, and decide that his/her Pitta is clearly out of balance.

Now it's your turn. Use the information from this chapter, and the prompts I have listed for you below, and write your personal plan. The most difficult task is to make a commitment, and getting started. Once you have it all written down, it becomes official and you will feel more inclined to move forward.

- *My intention* is:*

- *My goals* are:*
  1.

  2.

  3.

- *My Ayurvedic constitution is:*

- *The signs that my constitution is out of balance are:*
  1.

  2.

  3.

- *I will start my day with:*

- *New foods that I will include in my daily diet are:*
  1.

  2.

  3.

- *Foods that are not good for me and I am going to avoid are:*
  1.

  2.

  3.

- *Physical activities that I am going to do 3-4 times a day are (please include days, times of the day, and the amount of time you are committing to the activities):*
  1.

  2.

  3.

- *I will go to bed consistently at:*

- *Activities that I will include each week to find more joy and happiness are (e.g. visiting with friends, playing with kids, laughing more, listening to music, journaling):*
  1.

  2.

  3.

- *Once or twice a month I will treat myself with (e.g. getting a professional massage or acupuncture, attending a mini-retreat, going away for a day or two, attending a restorative yoga class):*

Visit your plan frequently to stay motivated. Modify the list as you start implementing the changes in your life. You will find that some of the commitments are easy and they quickly become your second nature, but some will require more time and discipline. To start, you can list only one goal, one food that you would like to add to your daily diet along with one food you plan to avoid, one physical activity, and one fun thing that you choose to do each week. With time you will keep adding things to your list and expanding your personal health and wellbeing plan.

*Intention is not the same as goal (read more about intention in chapter 1). The main difference between intention and goal is that intention refers to a present moment desire, whereas goal refers to a future achievement. You can think about the intention as a journey, and the goal as a destination.

Chapter 7

You Are What You Can Digest

One of the key areas of concern in Ayurveda is digestion. The type and quality of food that we eat is important, but even more crucial is how it is digested, absorbed, and eliminated. Instead of one diet for all, Ayurveda gives recommendations for each individual based on his or her constitution. However, there are a few universal suggestions, and one of them is eating seasonal foods. This makes a lot of sense to me because during the time when I was growing up in Poland the only way not to be hungry was to eat what nature was serving us, or what we were able to preserve and store for the winter. There is a lot of wisdom and health in this approach. Our bodies need to adapt to changes that happen every season. Somehow the Western society has decided that it does not matter if we eat berries shipped from California in the winter or grilled meat butchered in New Zealand in the summer. From the number of people that suffer from digestive issues, this method is not working very well.

We can receive great benefits from paying attention to the kinds of foods that grow, and are harvested during each season. In addition, observing animals (such as: foxes, deer, squirrels, and other animals living in the forests) and the kinds of food they eat can be helpful for understanding our own needs for example: animals eat certain foods to reduce dampness in the spring, and heat in the summer. They also prepare very well for cold winter months by eating more foods that build fatty insulation to stay worm and comfortable. By observing the eating behaviors of animals, we as humans, learn very helpful information on the types of foods that are best for us to eat during each season. Then we wouldn't need to try so many diets that make false promises, and in the long run don't deliver the best results. See the Resources in the back of the book for more information on a seasonal diet.

Our grandparents still remember that mealtime used to be a reason for celebration. People gathered around the table with their loved ones, and shared about their lives. In some cultures around the world, some people still continue this tradition. But in the Western world, we no longer have time to cook, to eat, and to celebrate! Some of the biggest mistakes leading to poor digestion and nutritional deficiencies are eating on the run, not chewing food properly, and eating while watching TV, driving, checking emails, and texting. Our digestive systems are not able to process food unless we are relaxed. Because eating on the run is stressful many people develop health conditions related to poor digestion. Ayurveda encourages everyone, regardless of his or her constitution, to eat slowly, breath deeply, relax and enjoy whatever is on the plate. It is known as mindful eating, but I call it "eating meditation". If you want to lose weight or find answers to your digestive problems, perhaps eating mindfully will help. Certainly, you will not only need to eat less, but will also assimilate your food better.

Our food is not as nutrient dense as it was hundred or even fifty years ago (which means that it is high in calories, but low in nutrients). Our soil is depleted from over-farming, and is contaminated with harmful chemicals from pesticides, air pollution, oil and gas production, and high levels of trash. In addition, the companies that manufacture unhealthy processed foods have convinced us through their advertisements, that we would be more productive if we didn't cook, but instead ate packaged foods or relied on restaurants and take-outs. I can tell you from my personal experience that this does not work! You can't be more productive if you are malnourished, and not feeling well. Ayurveda is accurate and clear—food is the first thing that we need to fuel the body and mind, to promote health, prevent disease, to be calm, and think clearly.

Several foods and spices are considered especially healthy in Ayurvedic cooking. They are nourishing to all three constitutions, easy to implement in a daily diet, and perfect to replace unhealthy choices. Most of these foods are also rich in nutrients and flavors so that only a small amount is needed to feel satisfied. Just remember, more is not always better. Below you will find the description and application of the foods that I have chosen for this chapter. I cook with them for my family, and I often recommend them to my clients.

Ghee is clarified butter, which means that the milk solids and buttermilk from the butter have been removed. Because ghee is free of lactose and casein, it is often a good choice for people with food allergies. It has a very high smoke point (it doesn't start burning until reaches 485 °F), which makes ghee one of the best fats for frying and sautéing. It is a staple in the Ayurvedic kitchen and medicine cabinet. It has been used as a carrier for ingesting herbs, a lubricating agent for the intestinal track, and a tool to detoxify the body. It is used to pull fat soluble toxins during the Ayurvedic cleanse called Panchakarma (read more about Panchakarma in chapter 12). Ghee nourishes, grounds, and supports the health of all three doshas.

Try this: Look for unsalted, organic and grassfed butter. Place the butter in a pan, and let it melt over medium heat. Once it has melted, reduce the heat and let it simmer for another 10-15 minutes. During that time you will notice foam forming on the top that needs to be removed with a spoon. Take the pan off the heat, for the butter to cool slightly, and then strain it thorough a strainer with a few layers of cheesecloth. Ghee does not have to be stored in the fridge, but it will last longer.

Coconut oil has been very popular lately, and some sources consider it "the healthiest oil on earth". It is great not only for cooking, but also for hair and skin care. It is cooling for the body and best used during the summer by all dosha types, but for Pitta all year round. (Coconuts grow in the tropical parts of the world and provide nourishment, hydration, and cooling properties to people and animals that cope with high air temperatures).

Try this: Add a tablespoon of raw and unrefined coconut oil to your morning oatmeal for a more satisfying breakfast.

Dates are rich and relatively heavy so having 2-3 a day is all you need. They are abundant in fiber, vitamins, and minerals. They are a great source of energy for the body. Their sweet and satisfying taste feeds the soul with peace and tranquility. Dates are balancing and pacifying for Pitta and especially Vata types.

Try this: Stuff a couple of dates with tahini or any nut butter, and roll them in coconut flakes for a healthy dessert or to conquer a sweet tooth attack.

Almonds are abundant in essential nutrients (vitamins, minerals, protein, and healthy fat), and they are also rich, so up to 10 a day is plenty. A good way to make almonds more digestible is to soak them overnight and remove the skin before eating (the skin is slightly toxic). In moderation, almond milk, almond butter, and soaked and peeled almonds, are recommended for pregnant women, children, and elders as well as all dosha types.

Try this: Instead of putting protein powder in your morning smoothie, soak several almonds overnight, remove the skin and blend them together with other ingredients.

Cow's milk in Ayurveda is considered one of the healthiest foods if digested properly. However, it is not the kind of milk that is usually served with school lunches. It needs to be non-homogenized, organic, and preferably raw. According to Ayurveda, milk should not be consumed with these tastes: sour, bitter, pungent, salty and astringent. That means that offering a glass of milk with dinner is usually not a good idea. The best way to consume milk is warm with added spices such as ginger, turmeric, cinnamon, cardamom, and black pepper for better digestion. (If you don't have access to raw milk, look for Organic Valley or Kalona brands that offer non-homogenized and VAT pasteurized milk with cream on top).

Try this: Warm a cup of milk (until it comes to a boil) with a pinch of any of these spices: cinnamon, cardamom, turmeric, ginger (fresh or powder), black pepper, and a couple of chopped dates. Add a teaspoon of ghee, and combine it with other ingredients. Sip slowly before going to bed. You can use any milk substitute if you are not able to tolerate cow's milk. This beverage is also known as "Golden Milk" due to the golden color of turmeric, but perhaps also from the amazing properties that come from the spices combined with milk. Golden Milk is soothing and grounding for any dosha, but especially for the Vata type during the cold winter months.

Honey is well known for its medicinal properties, but only raw honey should be consumed. According to Ayurveda, honey that is heated to a high-temperature changes its structure, and becomes hard to digest (it's OK to put it in hot tea, but not in cooking or baking). Honey is a warming type of food, and especially beneficial for Vata and Kapha constitutions.

Try this: On low heat, melt a few tablespoons of coconut oil. When the oil is melted, remove it from the heat, and add equal amounts of turmeric powder and raw honey. Add a pinch of black pepper, and mix all ingredients together to form a paste. Transfer the mix to a jar and eat a quarter to a half a teaspoon several times a day. I make this paste for my kids and give it to them when they are fighting colds and other infections. It works!

Lemons are purifying and nourishing. Fresh lemon juice mixed with water is one of the best and simplest ways to stimulate the digestion, and trigger a gentle detox. One of the most popular Ayurvedic morning rituals is sipping warm water with lemon juice before having coffee or breakfast. Because of their cooling and purifying properties, lemons are especially beneficial for Pitta and Kapha types.

Try this: Squeeze fresh lemon juice into a jug of filtered water. Add some maple syrup or honey to taste, and a few fresh mint leaves for a refreshing drink on a hot summer day.

Mung beans are particularly nourishing when mixed with basmati rice and cooked veggies. They are great for everyone, but especially for people that are sick, and need light wholesome food. They are full of protein, fiber, minerals, vitamins (especially vitamin B), and low in calories, sugar, and fat. Mung beans are pretty easy to digest; however they can be soaked overnight, and rinsed before cooking to make them even easier to assimilate for people with compromised digestion. Mung beans are healing and nourishing for all three dosha types.

Try this: On medium heat, melt a tablespoon of ghee. Chop some onions, carrots, potatoes, celery, parsnip, tomato, and any veggies that you like–put them into the pot. Add about 1 cup of rinsed mung beans, and fill the pot with filtered water or bone broth. Add spices such as turmeric, coriander, cumin, black pepper, and salt. Cook on low heat for about an hour. (Mung beans expand and absorb liquid during cooking, so make sure you keep adding water or bone broth.)

Fruits and veggies are also on the list of Ayurvedic superfoods. Fruits should be eaten ripe, in a season, and only between meals. Fruits make perfect snacks, and are a sort of a healthy version of fast food. Vegetables are always a part of a healthy lifestyle, Ayurvedic or not. Vegetables are truly healing due to their detoxifying, anti-inflammatory, and nourishing properties. However, if you are a Vata type, you might have difficulty digesting raw veggies. Cooking them lightly, making a vegetable juice or a smoothie, putting them in soups, mixing fresh salads with a lot of healthy oil (olive, sesame, avocado) will make veggies easier to digest and more enjoyable. Also, if you are not accustomed to eating a lot of veggies, increase the amount slowly, so your digestive system has a chance to adjust to the increase of fiber.

Ayurveda is known for using **herbs and spices** not only as medicine, but also as flavor enhancers. Cooking with certain spices makes food tastier (which eliminates the need for artificial flavors and fillers), and brings out powerful healing properties from all of the ingredients. It is exactly what the famous Hippocrates' quote says, "Let food be thy medicine and medicine thy food". Most of the herbs and spices are available in supplement form, but supplements are not as nearly beneficial due to relatively lower absorption.

Below you will find some examples of the spices that are commonly used in Ayurvedic cooking. Don't be afraid to experiment with them in your kitchen and discover their wonderful qualities.

Ginger can be used dry (in a powder form) or fresh (root). Both, powder and root, have a very strong taste. Ginger is known for helping with digestive problems such as nausea, indigestion, and gas, as well as the absorption and assimilation of food. Because of its anti-inflammatory and anti-viral properties, ginger is great for colds, respiratory diseases, arthritic conditions, and anything that lingers. You can use it in a marinade for meat or fish, add to stir-fried veggies, mix with salad dressing, add to soups and much more.

Turmeric has been making a lot of headlines lately. Used in India for thousands of years, now it is highly recommended by holistic practitioners in the West for just about anything including cancer, chronic pain, and the common cold. It's not easily absorbed in a supplemental form, therefore the best way to get the most benefits is to combine it with other spices (black pepper) and fat (ghee, coconut oil). While you are experimenting with turmeric in your kitchen, be aware of the orange color that stains very easily, and has a strong bitter taste that takes time to acquire. I hide turmeric in tomato sauce, bone broth, ground meat, scrambled eggs, and stir-fried veggies. If I have fresh turmeric root, I like to add a small piece to my morning veggie juice. I also add fresh ginger.

Cardamom is one of the spices found in chai tea. It not only tastes really good, but also it aids digestion and calms the nervous system. It was known in ancient Greek, Egyptian, and Roman cultures as an effective aphrodisiac. Try to remember this the next time when you order another cup of chai tea.

Cinnamon does not need a lot of introduction. It is well known for balancing blood sugar, but you might be surprised to learn that it also relieves coughs and colds as well as improves circulation and cognitive memory. One way to use it is in the morning with oatmeal. It also adds unique and delicious flavor to soups, stews, baked beans, hot chocolate, and French toast. It can be purchased in a powder form or sticks that can be easily removed at the end of cooking.

Coriander is a cooling type of herb, and is especially recommended for anyone with too much heat (inflammation) in the digestive system. It is detoxifying and helps in pulling out heavy metals. It is also used to relieve hot flashes, eliminate the root cause of allergies, and strengthen the immune system. In cooking, it mixes well with other spices, and adds flavor to meat dishes, grains, veggies, and beans.

Cumin not only makes beans a lot more digestible, if added while cooking, but it is also known as a medicine for reducing inflammation in the gut, and relaxing the colon. Cumin combines very well with other spices such as coriander, turmeric, black pepper, and garlic. It can be added to a variety of dishes including: soups, stews, casseroles, and all legumes.

Fennel seeds are known for their calming effect on the digestive system. Fennel tea is gentle enough that it's often recommended to give to babies for colic and tummy aches. Many Indian restaurants in the United States offer a bowl of roasted fennel seeds before meals to stimulate the appetite and to get the digestive enzymes ready to break down the food. It is also known to relieve menstrual cramps and PMS.

Try this: Bring three cups of filtered water to a boil. Add one teaspoon of each: coriander, cumin, and fennel seeds. Lower the temperature and simmer for 5-10 minutes. Strain and sip throughout the day to relieve stomach pain and indigestion. This beverage, also called CCF tea, can help with a natural and gentle detox.

It's important to know which foods are more nourishing than others, but until we learn how to listen to our bodies we won't know what we are able to digest, assimilate, and eliminate. Everyone is different. The growing number of people suffering from food allergies and sensitivities indicate that body awareness is key. This skill can be learned through regular yoga practice. In addition, moving through yoga poses (twists, forward bends, and back bends) stimulate the organs that are responsible for digestion. The recipe for a healthy digestion is pretty simple: choose the food that is right for you, move your body, and give yourself a chance to relax.

Chapter 8

"Do It Yourself" Ayurvedic Therapies

In addition to diet and nutrition, the Ayurvedic healing system offers many therapie
to support the body and mind. Some of them need to be performed or supervised b
an experienced practitioner, but some can be easily accomplished at home on a regula
basis with little financial investment. In Ayurveda, prevention is key. Most of thes
therapies are designed to keep the body and mind in balance. However, they can als
play a role in supporting conventional treatments for many common health problem
such as: stress, fatigue, chronic disease, and depression. There are many technique
(in addition to yoga, breathing exercises, meditation, and diet changes) that are wort
trying at home, and can be added slowly to your daily routine.

Dry Brush Massage is one of my favorite techniques. I do it almost every day befor
the shower. It takes only a couple of minutes, and it has many benefits if done regularly
The most visible benefits are: the smooth look of the skin (after gently removing dea
cells), improving circulation, and invigorating oil-producing glands. On a deeper leve
dry brush massage is excellent to help the body cleanse from toxins by stimulating th
lymph system—one of the most important ways our body detoxifies.

*Try this: Use a loofah, soft brush, or face cloth. Gently brush the skin moving towar
the heart. Start with the feet (soles and tops of the feet), and move from the heels an
ankles up the legs toward the torso using quick strokes. Then brush the arms movin
from the hands toward the armpits. Gently massage your belly moving in a circula
and clockwise direction, then reach behind to massage your back. Rub your hea
with your fingers. Move the dry brush on the neck, shoulders, and chest. Follow th
dry brush massage with a warm and relaxing shower or bath. For maximum benefit:
finish with massaging your skin with warm oil (before or during the shower).*

Self-Massage (*Abhyanga*) is another type of therapy recommended by nearl
every Ayurvedic practitioner. Besides the fact that it promotes softness of the ski
and preserves youthfulness, it helps to keep muscles, tissues and joints flexible an
healthy. The most important reason to do self-massage is to calm the nervous syster
and relieve stress. Self-massage is balancing for all constitutions, but is especiall
effective for grounding the Vata type during winter months. It's the power of touch
even if it is your own.

Try this: Pour some oil (sesame oil is usually recommended, but coconut or olive oil can be used as well) into a small jar, and immerse it in hot water to warm it up. Once the oil is warm, pour a little bit onto your palms. Begin by massaging your head (you can also start from the feet and work your way up), using your palms rather than your fingers. Apply more oil to your palms and your fingers to massage the face, back of the ears, and neck (back and front). Move downwards to the shoulder joints and arms. Use up and down motions on long muscles, and circular motions on shoulder joints, elbows, and wrists. Use circular motions around the nipples, and down strokes over the breastbone. Gently massage the abdomen using a clockwise motion. Reach behind to massage the back and spine with up and down motion. Massage legs vigorously with upward strokes toward the heart. Spend a little extra time massaging your feet: the tops, the bottoms, and around the toes. It is a good idea to spend a few minutes to relax, and allow the oil to absorb before a warm shower or a bath. If you don't have a lot of time, you can perform the self-massage while in a warm shower (remember that your feet are oily and slippery so be careful while stepping into the bath tub or shower).

Tongue Scraping is a quick and easy routine that can significantly improve your oral health. Many years ago, I was constantly suffering from gingivitis (gum inflammation). After trying many different protocols recommended by dentists, I discovered a tongue scraper. Ever since then, I have incorporated tongue scraping into my daily routine, and now I don't have any problems with my gums.

If your tongue is covered with a lot of coating, it means that your digestion is sluggish, because toxins, bacteria, and yeast accumulate on top of the tongue. This is why most of the Ayurvedic (and traditional Chinese medicine) practitioners always examine the tongue during a patient evaluation. Nowadays, conventional medicine admits that there is a connection between oral health and heart disease, as well as many other inflammatory health conditions.

Try this: Find a tongue scraping tool ($5-$10) in a local health food store or online. Use it in the morning and/or in the evening. Gently move the scraper from the back to the front of the tongue several times removing any coating that has accumulated.

Oil Pulling is an ancient technique that involves swishing a tablespoon of oil in the mouth. Similarly to tongue scraping, this therapy helps to improve oral health by removing toxins and bacteria from the oral cavity. In addition, swishing the oil for 5-20 minutes activates enzymes that are very good at pulling the toxins out of the blood. This is the main reason this therapy is recommended for oral and overall health.

Try this: In the morning, before you have any food or drink, use a tablespoon of goo quality, unrefined sesame, coconut, or olive oil. Put it in your mouth, swish it aroun and pull it through your teeth. Do it for 15-20 minutes (you can start with 5 minute and work your way to 20 minutes). Remember not to swallow the oil, and when you ar finished, spit it out in the trash (it has toxins), and rinse your mouth with clean wate.

Neti Pot is a container that resembles a small teapot, and is used for nose irrigatio to clear sinuses from mucus due to allergies, colds, sinus infections, and air pollutior Nose irrigation can be administered for chronic and acute conditions as well as to kee the nostrils clean. I use it throughout the entire winter.

Salt water can be drying on the delicate lining inside the nostrils, but there is an herba infused oil called Nasya, (or a couple of drops of sesame oil) that can be used after th neti pot rinse.

Try this: Look for a neti pot in a local pharmacy or health food store. Make a salin solution using warm distilled or sterilized water (boil water for 10-15 minutes an then cool it down); add a pinch of non-iodized salt. Bend over the sink and tilt you head to the side. Breathe through the mouth while pouring the water into the uppe nostril. After a few seconds, you will see the water coming down through the lowe nostril. Repeat on the other side. It might take a few tries before you figure it out fo yourself, but if my 9-year-old son can do it, you can do it, too. If you are using Nasy oil, lie down and put a few drops in each nostril.

Hot Water Bottle is a rectangular shaped rubber container, and a wonderful tool t use for comfort, relaxation, constipation, aches, pains, cramps, and belly aches. If use for pain relief, massage castor oil onto the painful area before placing on the wate bottle–making this therapy a lot more effective. A hot water bottle can also come i handy after overeating. Holding it on the belly for 20-30 minutes after eating is know to increase the production of hydrochloric acid necessary to break down food.

Try this: Most of the drug stores carry hot water bottles, so you should not hav trouble finding one (I got mine from Target). Once you have it, fill the bottle with hc water and lie down on the floor (or bed) with a large pillow under the knees, an the hot water bottle on your belly. If you need support for your neck, place a folde towel under your head. Relax your arms and shoulders, and breath deeply. Let th belly naturally move up and down as you inhale and exhale. Stay there for at least 1 minutes, and focus on relaxing, breathing, and letting go of any resistance.

Hot Water Therapy is simply drinking pure, boiled hot water throughout the day, but especially in the morning and 15-20 minutes before meals. In the morning, a glass of hot water helps to wake up the digestive system, and clean the body from toxins. Drinking water 30 minutes before meals turns on the digestive fire, which is a crucial component of good digestion. Sipping hot water during the day stimulates the lymph system and organs that are responsible for cleansing the body, and keeping the immune system working properly. According to some experts, hot water hydrates human cells much better than cold water. Proper hydration is vital in preventive health as well as healing. Hot water therapy doesn't cost anything, has no side effects, and therefore it is worth trying *(Douillard, Colorado Cleanse, 36)*.

Try this: Boil some filtered water in the morning, cool it down just enough so you don't burn yourself, and slowly drink the whole glass before drinking anything else or having breakfast. Pour the rest of the water into a thermos so it stays hot, and take it with you to work or school. Take sips every 15-20 minutes throughout the entire day.

Hydrotherapy is just a fancy name for taking a long bath in warm or hot water. It is known around the world for its relaxing and stress relieving properties. In Ayurveda, hydrotherapy is also considered a physical and spiritual cleansing ritual. One way or another, taking a warm bath feels really good, and helps with colds, congestions, joint and muscle pain, sleeping trouble, anxiety, and more.

Try this: Plan your day, so you have about half an hour to relax before you need to go to sleep. Fill the bathtub with warm water adding 2 cups of Epsom salts and a few drops of your favorite essential oil. Dim the lights, and turn on some soothing tunes. Before you jump into the tub, perform a dry brush massage, and self-massage with warm oil. While you are soaking in the water, remember to breathe deeply, relax the muscles, and calm the mind.

This chapter explains only some Ayurvedic "tricks and treats", but there are many more that the Ayurvedic healing system has been using for centuries. Let's not forget that Ayurveda has been around for thousands of years, which means that it is a well-proven system for health and wellbeing. With the growing popularity of yoga, learning Ayurvedic methods is the best next step to heal and help your wellbeing.

Part Three

PRACTICE: Practice Makes Anything Possible

Chapter 9

Lets Do It!

"Yoga is 99 % practice and 1% theory."

- Pattabhi Jois

Part One of this book explains what yoga is, where it comes from, and how it can influence your wellbeing. Part Two contains information about Ayurveda, and its connection to yoga, nature, and life in general. Perhaps the information about the Ayurvedic doshas has helped you to decide whether you are Vata, Pitta, or Kapha (or any combination of all three) to then be able to use this knowledge to have a better understanding of your health needs. However, having this wisdom is not going to change much in your life unless you act, and **do it now**. Don't wait until you are ready; it might not happen soon enough. Choose to use yoga and Ayurveda to become a part of your lifestyle, give it a try, see how it feels, and where it takes you. And remember that even though it's great to have goals and dreams, it's the journey that makes you stronger and opens up many possibilities.

Part Three of this book is designed to help you start your yoga practice, and make changes in your lifestyle according to your needs. If you already have an existing practice, it will give you new ideas and inspiration to continue. Changing habits and old patterns is not easy, and requires patience, discipline, and planning. You don't need to make the changes all at once, and I recommend that you don't. Make a plan and commit to it. Take one step at a time. Explore one pose before you move on to the next one. Add one superfood one week and sample another a week later. Think about which Ayurvedic therapy you would like to try first then when that becomes your routine, go for another one. If you can devote 10-15 minutes a day (the morning usually works best), do the practices you find are the most suitable and appealing to you such as: having a short yoga practice (see examples in Part Three of this book), seated or walking meditation, taking several conscious breaths, having a glass of warm water first thing in the morning, setting an intention for the day, and writing it down with a gratitude note. If you stick to your commitments, eventually you will crave more yoga practice, more foods that make you feel good, and more Ayurvedic methods

that work for your body and mind. By including Yoga and Ayurveda in your lifestyl
and noticing their benefits, you will change your life and positively influence the live
of those around you.

In the following chapters, I am going to map out some ideas for you to start you
yoga practice. Keep in mind that these are just ideas, and there is a lot more for yo
to explore further with taking various classes, finding different teachers, looking int
other resources, or talking to people that have practiced yoga for some time. Begi
with an intention and then listen to your breath, your body, and your intuition. Onc
you begin using your tools, with patience and discipline, you will be on your wa
toward making the practice your own. The way you do it is personal to you, becaus
it will be **Your Yoga**.

In the following chapters, you will find short practices and tips that can help situatior
that may currently be in your life. In addition to more specific practices, there are som
general sequences recommended by many teachers and practitioners. One of them
called Sun Salutations *(Surya Namaskara)*. It's a form of flow, moving with the breat
from one pose to another, and repeated as many times as needed. It's usually dor
at a vigorous pace, but the poses can be held for longer to slow down the pace. Su
Salutations are poses that can be done by themselves, or as a part of a longer practic
(often as a warm up or a way to let go of excess energy), usually practiced in th
morning or the earlier part of the day. On the next page you will find instructions o
how to practice Sun Salutations. When you find an opportunity, locate a class wher
you can become comfortable with each pose, and linking them together with the breat

Try this: Sun Salutations - Surya Namaskara

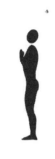

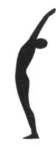
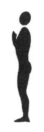

1. Natural breathing:
Mountain Pose

2. Inhale:
Raised Arms

3.Exhale:
Forward Fold

4. Inhale:
High Lunge

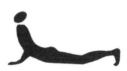

5. Exhale:
Downward Facing Dog

6. No breathing:
Caterpillar

7. Inhale:
Cobra

8. Exhale:
Downward Facing Dog

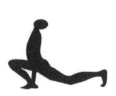
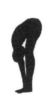
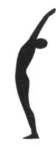
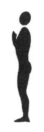

9. Inhale:
High Lunge

10.Exhale:
Forward Fold

11. Inhale:
Raised Arms

12. Exhale:
Mountain Pose

Chapter 10

Feeling Stressed?

Take a moment to observe your breath and your body language. If your breath i
short and choppy, that's an indication that you are stressed. If your chest is tigh
your shoulders are tense, your belly is gripping, and your jaw is clenching, you ar
definitely stressed out. Unless you are trying to escape from a lion or a car about to hi
you on a crosswalk, take a moment and relax. Have you already noticed that relaxin
is not always as easy as it sounds? Relaxing is a practice that requires awareness
commitment, and reliable tools such as deep breathing, meditation, visualization, an
movement.

Very often we are not aware of the stress, tension, and disconnection occurring in ou
bodies. In teaching yoga at a Rehabilitation Center for men and women, I becam
especially aware of the difficulty some people have with relaxation. Most of thes
people were on a probation program that required them to attend yoga classes. The
had very strong bodies, big muscles, and very little fear of taking on challenging pose
such as headstands or shoulderstands. They could hold the poses for as long as the
were asked to hold them. It seemed like an easy class to teach, but the challenge
began when we came to the end of the class with the final relaxation pose. My toug
students became lost, scared, and confused. Relaxing and letting go of tension was on
of the most difficult things for them to do.

*Try this <u>Stress Releasing Practice</u>: Stand up and feel your feet deeply rooting dow
into the ground in this deeply grounding posture–**Mountain Pose** (Tadasana). Clos
your eyes or keep your gaze fixed onto a point out into front of you. Take a breat
and notice if your breath is easily moving through your body or if it becomes "stuck
somewhere along the way. Don't force it, but rather invite your breath to come in an
out. Relax any parts of your body that might be tight. Inhale and lengthen the spin
by reaching up with the crown of the head, exhale and relax the shoulders down fron
the ears. Take a few breaths, focusing on the exhalation by making it twice as long a
the inhalation.*

*When you are ready, stretch your arms up above your head to come to **Upward Salut**
(Urdhva Hastasana) by relaxing the shoulders down and lifting the chest up into
gentle back bend. Bring the torso upright and slowly bend from the hips, bringin*

our hands down to the floor and letting your head hang while stretching your neck in *Forward Fold* (Uttanasana).

After several breaths in the Forward Fold posture, bend the knees, place your palms on the floor and step back into **Downward Facing Dog** *(Adho Mukha Svanasana)– keeping your hips high and heels low, as close to the ground as possible. Stay in this pose for 5-10 breaths.*

Bend the knees and place them on the ground. Keep the big toes close to each other, but the knees apart so that your abdomen has enough room to expand, and drop between the thighs during inhalations, while softening and retracting on exhalations. Stretch your arms over your head, and relax your hands, forearms, and elbows onto the ground. Feel your forehead touching the earth. Close your eyes, and continue breathing in **Devotional Pose** *(Bhaktasana).*

Finish your practice with **Corpse Pose** *(Shavasana), by lying down on the ground with your feet apart at the distance of your hips. Your arms are a few inches away from your torso with palms facing up. If you are in a place where you are not able to lay down on the floor, take a seat and keep your spine long with your sitting bones reaching down while the crown of your head reaches up. Keep your shoulders relaxed, and your head lightly floating on top of your neck. Whether you are in Shavasana or a seated position, close your eyes, and stay in the present moment for at least one minute observing your breath.*

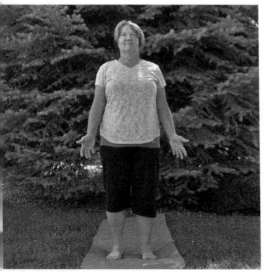

Mountain Pose

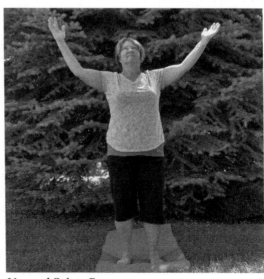

Upward Salute Pose

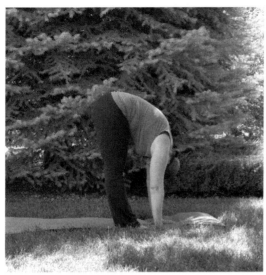

Forward Fold

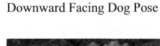

Downward Facing Dog Pose

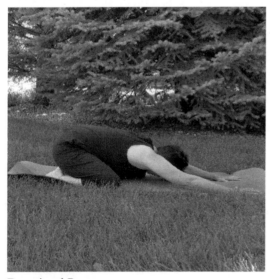

Devotional Pose

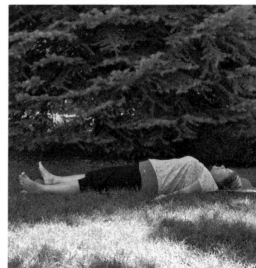

Shavasana

Shavasana is a very important part of your practice–please don't skip it. It's no only a final relaxation pose, but is an opportunity for your body to absorb and "digest" what you have just practiced. Corpse Pose is an opportunity to surrender, and let go o those things that you are not able to control; offering them to a higher power. Durin; this time, many practitioners experience a deep sense of freedom and release as wel as physical and emotional healing and restoration.

The above practice can be done anytime of the day. It is designed to help you become grounded and centered, slow down and regroup: to make the breath deeper and smoother, and to release tension. If you have extra time or if you need more rigorous exercise to burn off steam, do 1-10 sets of Sun Salutations (See Chapter 9 for instructions). Then come into Corpse Pose (Shavasana) or seated meditation. Another great way to end a stressful day is practicing a deeply restorative and stress relieving posture–Legs Up the Wall (please see Chapter 11 on how to do it).

For quick stress relief, try the following breathing technique that is accessible anywhere, at any time, and in any position (seated, standing, and reclined). The only two things that you need to know are how to breathe and how to count. Here you go: inhale through your nose and count to four, hold the breath and count to four, slowly exhale through your mouth and count to eight. Repeat 5-10 times and then breathe naturally. You can practice it throughout the day as many times as needed.

The following are examples of different yogic and Ayurvedic techniques that you might consider to stay balanced, grounded, and help you respond to stress in a sensible way.

Consider this:
- *Get up 15 minutes before your usual time. Start your day by setting an intention for the day and writing down a few things you are grateful for in your life.*
- *Perform one of these exercises or a combination: yoga, Tai Chi, mindful walking, and/or meditation.*
- *Do a self-massage before showering (see Chapter 8 for description).*
- *Take a break between 12:00 PM and 2:00 PM to clear your mind, and enjoy your lunch (that should be your biggest meal of the day).*
- *Consider having a bowl of warm soup in the winter, and a refreshing salad in the summer.*
- *Instead of another cup of coffee, consider having tea with cinnamon, cardamom, ginger, and a little bit of honey.*
- *At least once a week take a warm bath before going to bed (see Chapter 8).*
- *Go to bed no later than 10 PM.*
- *Limit the time you spend watching TV, searching the Internet, or following your Facebook friends.*
- *Spend as much time in nature as possible.*
- *Surround yourself with positive people and true friends.*

Now it is your turn. Try the yoga practice suggested in this chapter (or find a different one), and include the practice in your schedule–do it every day. Each week choose one or two things from the list of suggestions above. Try them and commit to including them in your daily routine. Work towards establishing a healthy lifestyle that incorporate yogic and Ayurvedic ideas. Notice any changes, shifts, and accomplishments in you life. **Be grateful** for everything that you have, and possibilities that you are about t discover. Enjoy yourself, and share your positive energy with other people.

You might already have a practice plan in your head, but your plan does not becom official until you have it on paper. Use the sample in Chapter 6 to help you develo, a personal plan, and then write your plan below. Each week write down a few thing that you are committing to doing and/or to changing in your daily routine.

My personal plan:

Chapter 11

Slowing Down the Aging Process with Yoga and Ayurveda

Almost everyone is interested in how to slow down the aging process. This is why the anti-aging industry is booming. So far no magic pill has been discovered, and no amount of money spent on cosmetics, procedures, or plastic surgeries will make the wrinkles disappear. If they do, it will only be a temporary solution. Preserving a youthful appearance does not have to be difficult or costly, but it does require commitment and determination. A good place to start is to learn and understand your unique constitution (see Chapter 6). To learn how to adjust your lifestyle according to your body type, and to maintain balance throughout your life.

Yoga can contribute to many youthful attributes that endure for a long time, beyond being concerned about wrinkles. These enduring characteristics are: mobility, balance, strength, flexibility, and overall health. There are poses that also support the youthful look of skin and body structure such as: **Inversions**–bring more blood and oxygen to the facial tissues, and reduce the presence of wrinkles. **Twists** and deep breathing are especially great for detoxification, and lymph flow to clear any skin impurities. **Forward bends**–relax the facial muscles, which may soften wrinkles. **Balance poses**– build strength and body awareness, which helps with keeping a good posture and reducing accidental falls. **Deep Breathing** and **Meditation** are great tools to minimize stress levels that contribute to premature aging. On a deeper level, yoga helps us to age gracefully especially when we accept the unavoidable changes in appearance that come naturally with aging.

*Try this <u>Anti-Aging Yoga Practice</u>: Take a few breaths standing in **Mountain Pose** (Tadasana), with feet at hip-distance apart, arms and shoulders down, chin retracted and the crown of the head reaching up. With each breath, lengthen the spine and become taller and stronger.*

*Bend from the hips to come to a **Forward Fold** (Uttanasana). Bring your hands or fingers down to the floor, bending your knees slightly, and letting your head hang. For a few breaths relax your facial muscles, and feel the skin separating from the bones. Take a deep breath, and twist as you exhale by walking your fingers to the left. Inhale, walk your fingers back in front of your feet. On the out breath walk them to the right, and then back in front of your feet. Bring your hands to your hips and rise up with* *elbows pointing up, keeping the spine long.*

*Step the left foot back about one leg length distance, with the hips facing forward, and bend the right knee. Inhale and stretch the arms up above the head. You are in **Warrior I** (Virabhadrasana I). Keep the shoulders down and away from the ears, feet pressing down to the floor, with the front knee stable above the heel, and the kneecap tracking the second toe.*

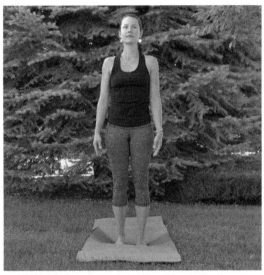

Mountain Pose

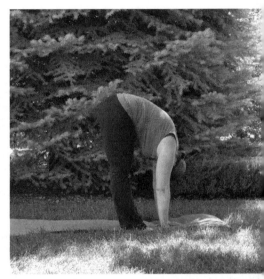

Forward Fold

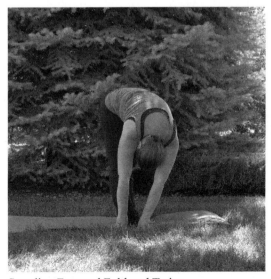

Standing Forward Fold and Twist

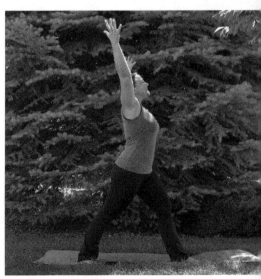

Warrior I Pose

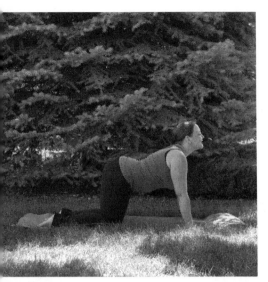

Cow Pose

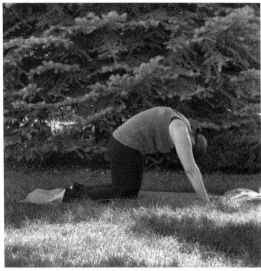

Cat Pose

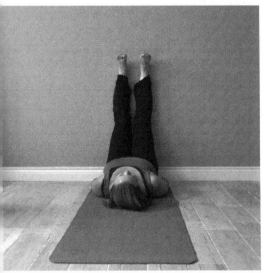

Legs Up the Wall Pose

*After a few deep breaths, step the left foot forward to meet with the right one, and repeat Warrior I on the other side. Come back to Mountain pose by stepping the right foot forward. Find your balance. When you are ready, bend from the hips, and fold forward. Then bend the knees, place them on the ground, and come to all fours. Inhale, lift the sitting bones up, arch the spine, and lift the head up; exhale, curl the tailbone, round the spine, and relax the head down. Go through this **Cat** pose and **Cow** pose sequence several times. Then come back to having a neutral spine.*

*Finish your practice, in my favorite pose, **Legs Up the Wall** (Viparita Karani), which is a deeply relaxing restorative inversion. Sit sideways with one hip near a wall. Swing your legs up the wall while you slowly bring your back down to the floor (use your hands and forearms to recline). Having your hips higher than your heart will make this pose a deeper inversion. To accomplish a deeper inversion, you can place a tightly folded blanket a few inches away from the wall, and then recline down with the blanket under your sacrum. You might also need some support under your head such as a small pillow or a folded towel. A good* *amount of time to spend in this pose would be 5-15 minutes. This pose can be a part o almost any practice or done alone.*

If you have extra time, before you do the Legs Up the Wall pose, I highly recommen doing a few sets of Sun Salutations.

Consider this:
- *Limit your sugar intake (especially pastries or products made from white flou sweet drinks including fruit juices, canned and dry fruit, cereals, milk shakes, ic cream, jams, preserves, marmalades, instant gravies, candies, and milk chocolate,*
- *Get at least 8 hours of sleep every night.*
- *Stay hydrated. Consider Hot Water Therapy during the cold months (see Chapte 8 for more details).*
- *Attend to any digestive problems that might be related to your constitution imbalances (more in Chapter 6).*
- *Get enough healthy fat in your diet such as ghee, sesame oil, olive oil, or cocon oil (see Chapter 7).*
- *Include plenty of fresh fruit and veggies in your diet.*
- *Move your body! Include: yoga practice (see the example above), Tai Chi, walkin biking, swimming, or anything that you like, but don't overdo it. Excessive exercis speeds up aging.*
- *Consider the dry brush technique and/or self-massage before showering (se Chapter 8).*
- *Instead of cosmetics use coconut oil as a moisturizer, rose water (available in mos of the Indian or Middle Eastern stores), or Aloe Vera juice as a toner.*
- *At least once a week take a warm bath (see Chapter 8).*
- *Go to bed before 10 PM.*

By using gentle and effective solutions offered by Yoga and Ayurveda, you can remai healthy and beautiful. As a matter of fact, YOU ARE! Just let your natural beaut come out and it will last for the rest of your life. With age, your beautiful soul neve gets wrinkled, but flourishes instead.

You might already have a practice plan in your head, but your plan does not becom official until you have it on paper. Use the sample in Chapter 6 to help you develop personal plan, and then write your plan on the other page. Each week write down few things that you are committing to doing and/or to changing in your daily routine

My personal plan:

Chapter 12

Detox Anyone?

To stay strong and healthy, we need to make sure our bodies and minds cleanse on a daily basis, so toxins don't accumulate and eventually make us sick or crazy. More and more people are realizing that they need to detox. Many people often choose programs or formulas they find in health food stores or online. In my opinion, any detox program or any cleansing formula should be based on an individual's needs, constitutional type, and supervised by an experienced practitioner. Besides dieting and fasting, detoxifying needs to occur at the time of the year when the body naturally wants to purge impurities (spring and fall). Cleansing is most effective during the time of life when an individual is ready to let go of physiological and emotional burden while also being able to relax and rest.

Ayurveda offers a therapy called *Panchakarma*. It is one of the most sensible cleanse I have tried. It has been recommended for thousands of years by many Ayurvedic and yogic therapists. It is gentle, safe, and effective. It is also healing, rejuvenating, balancing, and deeply relaxing. Panchakarma usually occurs during three, five or seven-day periods depending on an individual's needs. It includes a particular diet (mainly a dish called *kitchari*), *oleation* (taking ghee on an empty stomach to access toxins on a cellular level), gentle yoga, oil massage (*Abhyanga*), and other treatment performed by an Ayurvedic therapist.

Our bodies need to detox efficiently on a daily basis to support the lymphatic system, gastrointestinal system, liver, kidneys, lungs, and skin. When our bodies detoxify efficiently, our systems do the hard work of getting rid of anything that doesn't serve us. However, there are a few reasons why we are not doing so well in this department. In the last fifty years, we have been exposed to a lot more toxins than ever before. It takes a very strong detox system to be able to get rid of all of the junk we absorb from the air, soil, water, cosmetics, processed foods, chemically treated household goods, and many other sources of toxins. The type of food that is currently popular generates a lot of metabolic waste. Our world has become chronically stressful, and when an individual is in a constant state of stress, her/his body does not cleanse very well because it is using all of its power to cope with stressful circumstances. Our lives have become so "convenient" that we don't have to move our bodies unless we choose to do so. Every day we make choices to either live with a positive attitude ınd abundance of energy, or to simply get through the day using the same patterns hat keep us from being healthy, happy, and fulfilled. These choices are neither easy nor quick to implement, but with some guidance, discipline, and determination they become a part of who we are, our constitution, and our DNA; choices that we can enjoy during our lifetimes, and pass on to the future generations.

One of the best ways to stimulate the internal organs and systems is to include some form of exercise in a daily routine. Yoga is excellent at addressing many areas where we might be struggling, and therefore not detoxing well. Yoga brings awareness to how we really feel, and helps to bring us clarity of mind as to what to do about it. A regular practice helps to keep the stress level down; deep breathing cleanses the system from metabolic and environmental gases. Many poses like inversions, twists, and forward bends stimulate the internal organs to work and detox more effectively. Your practice doesn't have to take much time, simply a few minutes of meditation, deep breathing, and asana will not only cleanse your body, but also help your mind to let go of many emotional toxins that contribute to your overall physical health.

Try this Detoxifying Yoga Practice: Start in **Easy Pose**–*a crossed-legged seated position. Bring awareness to the breath and body while slowing down the vortex of the mind. After several deep breaths, interlace the fingers in front of you, reverse the clasp and stretch both arms up (keep the elbows bent if necessary). Reach with the palms and the crown of the head up. Breathe into the left side of the ribcage as you gently bend to the right, and then breathe into the right side of the ribcage and bend to the left. Release the clasp and place your hands in front of your legs. Walk your fingers forward, fold from the hips by keeping the spine long and sitting bones on the floor. Come back up, cross your legs with other leg on top and fold forward again. Bring the torso upright. Inhale and stretch the arms to the sides (parallel to the floor); exhale, twist to the right starting from the navel. Inhale, come back to center. On the outbreath, twist to the left. Come back with the front of the body facing forward. Extend your right leg in front of you while bending the left knee and placing the sole of the left foot against the right thigh. Inhale, lift the arms up; exhale, hinge from the hips and bend over the right leg into* **Head to Knee** *posture (Janu Sirsasana). Place your hands on the extended leg or on the floor. After five breaths, stretch your arms in front of you; using the strength of your core, bring the torso upright. Repeat on the other side.*

*Come onto all fours and then lift your knees and hips up into **Downward Facing Do** (Adho Mukha Svanasana). Keep the hips high, and heels as close to the ground a possible–press the front of the body towards the front of the legs, and the back of th legs toward the floor. Stay in this pose for 5-10 breaths.*

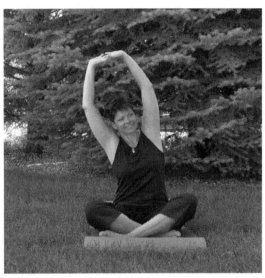

Easy Pose

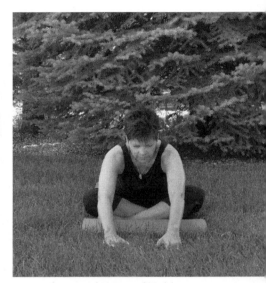

Crossed-Legged Forward Fold

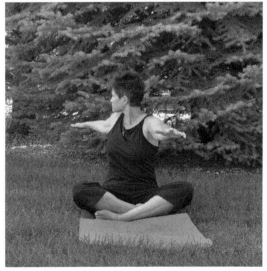

Side Bend

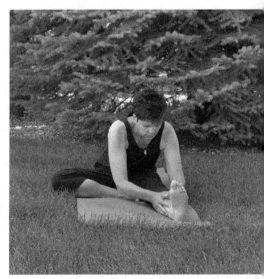

Head to Knee Pose

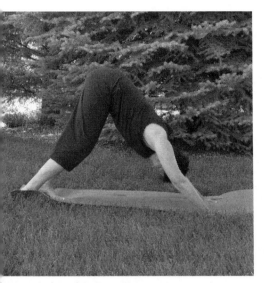

Downward Facing Dog Pose

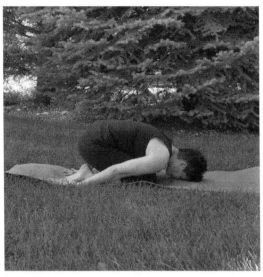

Child's Pose

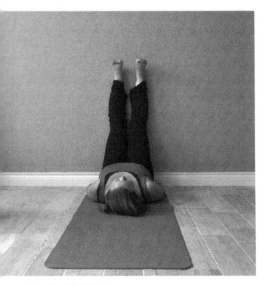

Legs Up the Wall Pose

*Bend your knees, bring your head down to the floor, arms and hands alongside the shins–settle into **Child's Pose** (Balasana). Keep your feet and your knees together, your abdomen resting on top of your thighs. Close your eyes, and feel your forehead touching the earth. Continue to breathe deeply. When you are ready, unroll your spine, and lie down with your back on the floor. Stretch your arms to the side (into a letter "T"), bend your knees; keep your feet on the floor and your legs together. On the outbreath bring your legs to the side as close to the floor as possible, and breathe deeply, flushing the toxins from the organs in the abdominal cavity. After a few breaths, lift your legs back up and slowly lower them to the other side.*

*Finish your practice in a restorative and lymph-stimulating pose–**Legs Up the Wall** (Viparita Karani). Bring a mat or a blanket close to the wall. Sit sideways with one hip a few inches away from the wall, and swing your legs up the wall; bringing your* *back down to the floor (use your hands and forearms to recline), and your buttoc. as close to the wall as possible. For a deeper inversion with the hips higher than th heart, you can place a tightly folded blanket a few inches away from the wall, and the recline down with the blanket under your sacrum. You might also need support und your head such as a small pillow or a folded towel. A good amount of time to spe in this pose would be 5 to 15 minutes. This pose can be a part of almost any practi or done alone.*

If you have extra time, before you do the Legs Up the Wall pose, do at least one s of Sun Salutations, but go through the poses slower, and hold each of them for a fe breaths.

Consider this:
*   *Avoid any food that is taxing on your detox system such as: products with add sugar, white flour, processed foods, anything artificial (flavors, colors, sweeteners also avoid GMOs, commercial dairy, and meats from factory farms.*
*   *Eat enough food that contains fiber: fruits, veggies, whole grains, seeds, and bea (especially mung beans).*
*   *Have an early light supper, and avoid snacking after your last meal.*
*   *Eat slowly and mindfully to avoid overeating.*
*   *Start using herbs and spices especially: ginger, cumin, turmeric, coriander, a fennel. Drink a few cups a day of CCF tea (See Chapter 7) to stimulate detoxificatio.*
*   *Drink plenty of clean water. Consider Hot Water Therapy during the cold seaso (see Chapter 8).*
*   *Address any digestive problems that might be related to your constitution. imbalances (see more in Chapter 6).*
*   *Move your body! Consider yoga practice (see the example above), Tai Ch walking, biking, swimming, or anything that you like, and keep it simple.*
*   *Consider the dry brush technique and/or self-massage before showering (s Chapter 8 for details).*
*   *Take a hot bath with Epsom salts as often as possible (see Chapter 8).*
*   *Remove toxic build up with tongue scraping, oil pulling, and neti pot (look f details in Chapter 8).*
*   *Get plenty of sleep. Go to bed before 10 PM.*
*   *Begin working on releasing emotions that cause toxic build-up in your mind a body.*
*   *Some relationships are more toxic than the food you eat and the air that y breathe. Take an inventory of your relationships.*

There is a lot you can do to get your body to cleanse, and function very well. Your body is designed to cleanse. Slowly start implementing yogic and Ayurvedic ideas until they become part of your life. You will see a big difference in how you feel, and healthy choices will be easy to make.

You might already have a plan in your head, but your plan does not become official until you have it on paper. Use the sample in Chapter 6 to help you develop a personal plan, and then write your plan below. Each week write down a few things that you are committing to doing and/or to changing in your daily routine.

My personal plan:

Chapter 13

Are You Sleepless?

The latest statistics show that sleeping problems are very common, and the reasons ar
not always as romantic as those that we have seen in the popular movie, *Sleepless i.
Seattle*. Most adults are not getting the recommended 7-8 hours of sleep, neither ar
school-age children who need 10-11 hours to be healthy, sharp, productive, and happy
Sleep is necessary for the body and mind to rest, rejuvenate, detox, and heal.

In the world of conventional medicine many sleeping disorders are often being treate
with medications. In some cases this might be necessary, but most sleeping problems ca
be addressed with simple lifestyle changes. Very often stress and anxiety are the reason
for being awake at night. Sleeplessness can create a vicious cycle, and even generat
more stress and more anxiety. In Ayurveda, any constitutional imbalances (see Chapte
6 for more information) can disturb a good night's sleep. A decent understanding of th
individual body type, and how to care for it, can serve as a solution to many sleeples
nights.

According to Dr. John Douillard, Ayurvedic Doctor and a founder of Life Spa in Boulde
Colorado, one of the reasons people do not sleep well is simply because they are too tirec
It sounds counter-intuitive, but it does make sense. I've had this experience many time
after a day of intense mental work (often using technology), and sitting for extende
periods of time. On the other hand, I don't remember ever having trouble sleeping afte
gardening, hiking, or swimming in the ocean. Even a short amount of time performin,
healthy physical activities during the day can make a big difference in the quality o
sleep later at night.

There are two different types of practices I recommend that will make a big difference i
the quality of your sleep. One is more vigorous, and performed in the morning or earl
in the day. The other one is a restorative practice that works best if performed shortl
before bedtime. The first practice is as simple as doing a few sets of Sun Salutations (se
Chapter 9 on how to do it), or taking a yoga class such as Vinyasa, Ashtanga, Powe
or a gentler and effective styles such as Hatha, Anusara, or Iyengar (See Chapter 3 fo
descriptions). However, walking, jogging, swimming, playing ball, biking or hiking wil
do the trick, and help you sleep well. The second practice is Restorative Yoga–a deepl
relaxing practice that helps unwind, and prepare the body and mind for deep rest.

Try this <u>Restorative Practice for Better Sleep:</u>   Before you start, find a towel, two blankets, a yoga mat (if you have one), and a chair. Roll one blanket into a thick tube, and the other one into a thin long tube. Sit on the floor with the long tube behind you, and the thick one under your knees. Using your hands and elbows slowly recline down. Adjust the long tube so it's directly under your shoulder blades, and your arms and shoulders are resting on the floor above the tube. If you feel like your head is falling back, use a towel under your head and neck. Stay here for at least 5 minutes relaxing and breathing deeply.

When you are ready, use your elbows, forearms, and hands to lift up your upper body. Come to a crossed-legged position with the chair right in front of your legs (if you need a modification, stretch your legs under the chair). Place your elbows and forearms on top of the chair with hands reaching for opposite elbows. Bend from the hips and place your forehead on top of your forearms. Stay in this posture for at least 5 minutes. Then slowly lift your spine to raise back up.

Keep the chair in front of you, lay with your back on the floor (support your head with the towel underneath if necessary), lift your legs, and place your calves and feet on the chair. Adjust the position, so that your legs from your knees to your feet are resting on the chair (if you are practicing in the bedroom, you can use your bed instead of the chair, or choose the Legs Up the Wall posture explained in Chapter 11). You can stay in this posture as long as you like (at least five minutes) while breathing deeply, relaxing the muscles, and letting go of any tension.

Slowly push the chair away and bring your legs to the floor. Place your hands on your abdomen, inhale and feel your belly rising. Then exhale—watch your abdomen retract, and sink closer to your spine. Take several breaths before slowly coming back up.

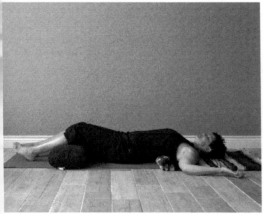

Mountain Brook Pose

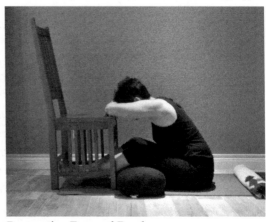

Restorative Forward Bend

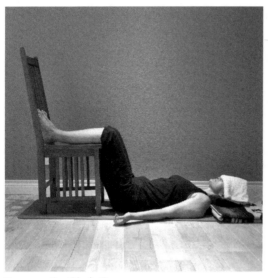 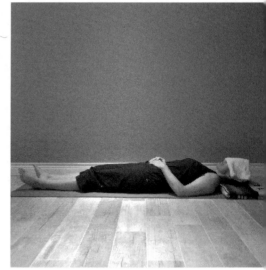

Legs on the Chair Pose   Shavasana

After the restorative practice described above, you should be able to fall asleep much faster, and sleep much better through the night. However, if you have had trouble sleeping for quite some time, it might take several days or weeks for the mind to stop interfering with your rest, and for the body to learn to relax. It might require more effort and more than one lifestyle change for you to be able to sleep well again. Whatever it takes, it's definitely worth it. You will look forward to going to bed at night, and waking up rested in the morning ready for a new day. After a good night's sleep, you will face your new day with energy, and the confidence necessary to make a difference in your life while also positively influence someone else's life as well.

Consider this:
- *Keep your dinner light, and eat it early.*
- *Avoid alcohol and caffeine in the evening. Instead, have a cup of warm Golden Milk (look for the recipe in Chapter 7).*
- *Before bed, do a self-massage and then take a warm bath (see Chapter 8).*
- *If you have trouble falling asleep because your mind is analyzing events from the entire day, keep an evening journal, and write down what bothers you. Then close the journal, take a deep breath and say to yourself: "Tomorrow is another day".*
- *Go to bed (optimally before 10 PM), and get up at the same time every day.*
- *Keep your bedroom dark at night, but get plenty of light during the day. Try to get some sunshine and fresh air during the day.*
- *Keep all electronics, including the TV, out of the bedroom.*

- *Try not to use the computer or watch TV, at least, one hour before bedtime. Instead, read a book or listen to music.*
- *Consider meditation or other techniques such as: deep breathing or visualization to work with stress in your life.*

Tomorrow is another day, and another opportunity to solve the problems that might be keeping you awake, but tonight is the night to sleep better. Look around your bedroom and figure out what you can change to create a more relaxing atmosphere. Read the list of suggestions above to see what you can try tonight to get yourself on track toward more restful nights.

You might already have a plan in your head, but your plan does not become official until you have it on paper. Use the sample in Chapter 6 to help you develop a personal plan and then use the space below to write your plan. Each week write down a few things that you are committing to doing and/or to changing in your daily routine.

My personal plan:

Chapter 14

Lose Weight and Feel Great!

Whether you are trying to lose a few stubborn pounds or you're truly overweigh
you probably already know—you are not alone. You might've already tried differer
diets or weight loss programs, and perhaps you have learned that most of them don'
work. You might've even lost weight, but gained it back later. Even though it a
seems difficult, and in some cases it is: maintaining healthy weight does not have t
be complicated. The Yogic and Ayurvedic logical approach to health and wellnes
makes it easy to understand conditions and circumstances for healthy weight, and hov
to maintain it throughout life.

There are several reasons you might be having trouble letting go of those extra pound
you have been carrying around such as stress, lack of healthy activity, bad nutritior
eating the wrong foods at the wrong times, hormonal problems, or other health relate
issues that create constitutional imbalances, and lead to weight gain (or loss) or disease

The best place to begin is having a good understanding of your constitutional bod
type (read more in Chapter 6), and an accurate perception of what healthy weigh
means for you. If you are a Kapha type, it is not natural or healthy for you to look lik
a Vata type, or if you are a Vata type you will not look like a Pitta type, unless yo
are out of balance. Find out who you truly are: your strengths and weaknesses, hov
to nourish and nurture your body, and how to love yourself unconditionally. Slowl
you will be able to let go of anything that does not serve you anymore—contributing t
your weight problem.

*Try this Yoga Practice for Healthy Weight: Start in **Hero Pose** (Virasana) sitting dow
on the floor with hips between your heels and knees together (use a block or a rolle
blanket under your sitting bones if it is challenging for you to bring them down t
the floor). If Hero Pose is not for you, come to a cross-legged position, or any seate
posture. Relax your muscles, lengthen your spine by reaching the crown of the hea
up, and let your breath become naturally deeper, longer, and smoother. Stay here fo
several breaths.*

*Then come to all fours, and do a few rounds of **Cat** and **Cow** postures: inhale, lift th
sitting bones up, arch the spine, and lift the head up; exhale, curl the tailbone, roun*

he spine, and relax the head down. Come back to a neutral spine (flat back), shift your hips to the left, and look over the left shoulder (make a "C" shape out of your spine) then turn your hips to the right, and look over the right shoulder. After a few rounds, lower the front of the body to the floor, keeping your hands under your shoulders.

Come to **Cobra Pose** (Bhujangasana): inhale, hug the elbows in, lengthen the spine by reaching the crown of the head forward, and slowly peel your head, shoulders, chest, ribcage, and belly off the floor; exhale, slowly lower your ribcage, chest and head down to the floor. Repeat this 3 more times with at least one breath between the postures. On the last one hold the posture for 3 long breaths before you come back down to the floor, then rest for several breaths.

Bring your hands under your shoulders, press your palms to the floor and lift your hips up into **Downward Facing Dog** (Adho Mukha Svanasana). "Walk the Dog" by bending one knee at the time, and letting the opposite heel of your foot stretch toward the floor. Slowly straighten both knees back into Downward Facing Dog and bring the heels closer to the floor. Hold the pose for a few more breaths. Walk your feet forward between your hands, and come to **Forward Fold** with your knees bent, head hanging between your upper arms and fingers touching the floor. Take several deep breaths.

Slowly bring your hands to your hips, bend your knees and lift your upper body coming into **Chair Pose** (Utkatasana). Bring your palms together in front of the chest. Inhale, and as you exhale slowly twist to the left from the hips by moving the right elbow towards the left knee (if it is within your ability, bring the right elbow to the outside of the left knee). Inhale, come back to center. Exhale, twist to the other side. Come back to center and lift up to **Mountain Pose** (Tadasana). After a breath or two, lie down in **Corpse Pose** to finish your practice while staying present, and breathing naturally.

I highly encourage you to include a few sets of Sun Salutations (See the instructions in Chapter 9) in your daily practice. You can hold each posture for 2-3 breaths, but when you get more comfortable, follow the breath, and get the momentum going. Sun Salutations make a great work out to detox, to energize, and to burn unwanted fat while focusing on the breath and the body-mind connection.

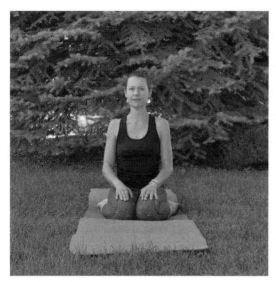

Hero Pose

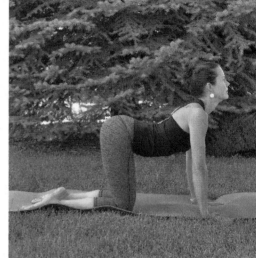

Cow Pose

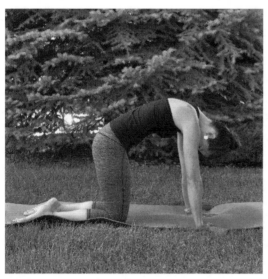

Cat Pose

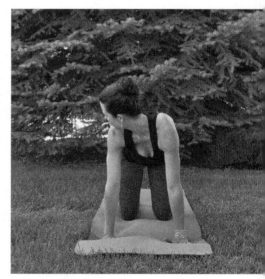

Spinal "C" Shape

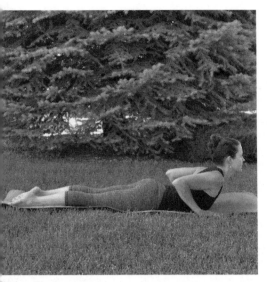

Cobra Pose

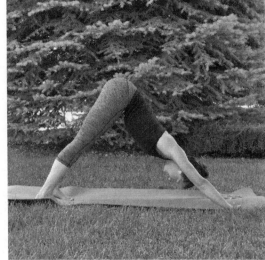

Downward Facing Dog Pose

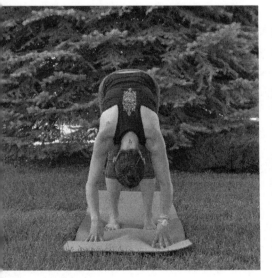

Forward Fold

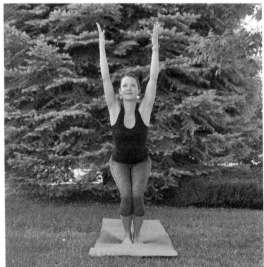

Chair Pose

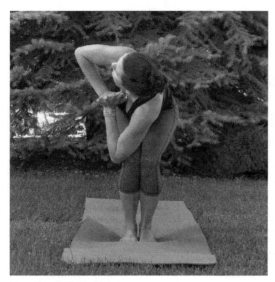

Revolved Chair Pose

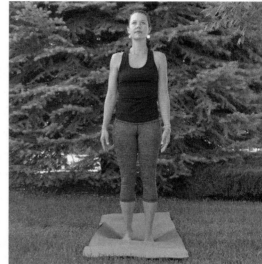

Mountain Pose

Consider this:
- *Start your day with a big glass of warm water with fresh lemon juice.*
- *Make sure that you have daily bowel movements. Eat enough foods that contai fiber: fruits, veggies, whole grains, seeds, and beans (especially mung beans).*
- *Have three meals a day at regular times and avoid snacking between them.*
- *Eat slowly and mindfully to avoid overeating.*
- *Stay away from sugar (natural or artificial) including white flour products, swee beverages, desserts, processed foods.*
- *Try to take a brisk walk after each meal (or any meal).*
- *Spice your food up with ginger, cumin, turmeric, coriander, black pepper an cinnamon (see Chapter 7).*
- *Drink plenty of plain filtered water (or water with lemon and ginger) throughou the day.*
- *Move as much as you can and break a sweat. Consider doing a yoga practice (se the example above), walking, biking, swimming, or anything that gets your bod moving. Do something every day*
- *Consider using the dry brush technique before the shower or bath (see Chapter 8)*
- *Remove toxic build up with tongue scraping, oil pulling and neti pot (look fo details in Chapter 8).*
- *Get plenty of sleep. Go to bed before 10 PM and get up no later than 6 AM.*
- *Keep a journal. Write what you have accomplished today, and the goals you hav for the future to keep going on your journey. Be grateful for every step along th way.*

Find a support system that will keep you encouraged and accountable. It is more fun to practice with others, and you are more likely to succeed if you are not doing it alone.

Even though your goal might be to lose weight, there are many other benefits that come from changing how you take care of yourself. These changes will help you to accomplish your main goal, and open up a whole new world where you can see things from a different perspective. Feeling better physically and emotionally will make it much easier for you to stay on the path of permanent weight loss, and help you to experience long lasting wellness and happiness. Give it a try, and you will never want to go back!

You might already have a plan in your head, but your plan does not become official until you have it on paper. Use the sample in Chapter 6 to help you develop a personal plan and then write your plan below. Each week write down a few things that you are committing to doing and/or to changing in your daily routine.

My personal plan:

Chapter 15

Listening to Your Heart, and to the Wisdom of My Students

In the previous chapters, I gave you the tools and encouragement to take charge c
your health and happiness. Changing your life means changing your old habits, an
this requires discipline, commitment, patience, and courage. It's never too late nor to
early to begin a new path toward leaving a healthy lifestyle that will serve you for th
rest of your life. Every breath you take is a gift, and every heartbeat is another chanc
to make your life more meaningful. Now is the time to stop rushing. Take a breath an
listen to your heart–it will tell you what to do and how to do it.

If you continue to have any doubts about whether yoga is worth your efforts, pleas
read the testimonials below. My students in Colorado and Alaska have shared thei
experiences, and have described what yoga practice has done for them. Even thoug
their experiences with yoga practice may vary, they have one thing in common: the
show up and they practice regularly.

*"Hatha Yoga Has Changed My Life. When I started taking Hatha Yoga classes som
17 years ago, I had no idea what I was in for. I had no concept about how disconnecte
I was from my body and spirit. I first noticed how uncomfortable I was doing basi
poses. This discomfort was from having an abusive childhood. I felt like I had been i
a permanent 'fetal position', and I was unable to relax my body at all. Slowly I starte
to crave the connection with a relaxed body and mind. I started to feel peacefu.
Gradually, I have blossomed into healing in all areas of my life over the years. Thank
to all of my yoga instructors."*

- Mary C., Colorad

***

*"I always feel refreshed and energized after taking a yoga class. It perfectly puts m
head and body in a place where I can have a wonderful day."*

- Barbara S., Colorad

I had been injured, and was seeing a chiropractor one to three times a week over the last year. After the first few yoga classes with Urszula, I returned to the chiropractor, and he said: 'Whatever you're doing, keep it up. I don't want to see you back for a whole month'. Since then I have become optimistic about my recovery!"

- Jesse C., Alaska

***

"Yoga has helped me stand taller and straighter, as witnessed by some of my friends. I can trim my toenails more easily since starting yoga (smile)."

- Ann F., Colorado

***

"I originally tried yoga as a tool to maintain my balance and stability. I was watching my mother and older relatives lose their balance too easily, and wanted to do something to avoid that as long as possible. I found yoga to be much more. I was surprised at the effort it took originally, and as a result learned quickly that it was not a sissy sport. In my early days of yoga, I enjoyed an improved golf game. It helped me attain a greater turn, and more stable footing. I now find that the regimen of attending yoga twice weekly greatly improves my calmness, and allows me to better manage any anxieties I experience. I have never seen a grumpy person leave a yoga class."

- Mike F., Colorado

***

*"I am Dan and would like to tell you why I do yoga.
#1 is to be able to play and enjoy my two grand kids.
#2 is to be able to compete at higher levels in several sports.*

I find that yoga helps me with balance and strength. I use those skills when I play with my two and four year old grand kids. I can only TRY to keep up with them, but by being in good shape I can spend more time with them and not be completely wiped out. Yoga also helps me with flexibility which is important to me because the more flexible I am the better my golf swing is. I play in national golf tournaments, and the more flexible I am the more I can compete against guys half my age.

My first priority with yoga is to learn to control my breathing. It really helps in facing stressful situations, and it also helps when I am playing in a tournament with a lot of the line. Breathing helps me focus which is critical in being a successful athlete. There are times when I must block out ALL distractions which could be anything from noise fear or even weather."

- Dan R., Colorado

***

"I started yoga 13 years ago to add flexibility to my strength training. Soon after, became quite ill from the side effects of a prior brain tumor hemorrhage. Yoga saw m through years of healing that I know would have been impossible without the physica emotional and endocrinological benefits of my practice. In addition to the healing, can look back and see the growth of joy in my life that accompanied my devotion practice. I never would have thought so much was possible when I took that first clas but then that is the beautiful serendipity of Grace, isn't it? As my teacher says, 'Set th sail and Grace will fill it'."

- Jane R., Alask

***

"My yoga class has given me renewed balance and flexibility in my life. I fee energized after a gentle yoga class with the meditative smooth flowing routine an good instructions."

- Sherry C., Colorado

***

"When I began my Yoga practice two years ago, I had no idea the benefits it woul provide to my body and mind. I had a tremendous amount of stress in my life, whic was negatively affecting my health.

Now, I have finally achieved inner peace. I have experienced a state of bliss tha has changed my daily life. Life occurs now at slower pace. I have an awareness everything around me that I didn't have before. I have better physical, mental, an spiritual health.

The Yoga asanas, or postures have made my body stronger and more flexible. The postures are so gentle and relaxing that they make a connection with my mind. As we go through the movements in class, I also feel a connection to fellow students. A peaceful energy can be felt in the room where we practice. At the end of a class, the Shavasana pose promotes a sense of wellbeing, which helps me to go forward in my life with inner peace."

- Debbie, Colorado

***

"Yoga is a huge part of my life. As an avid meditator, I am constantly working to establish a union of soul and spirit; yoga brings about a state of even-mindedness that surely leads to that union. I have been dealing with a health condition that has resulted in muscle weakness and balance issues. Regular yoga practice has helped immensely."

- A.R., Colorado

***

"In a sentence, yoga is helping me save my life. I know it's working on all levels, including body, mind, and spirit, because the other week as I was dropping my four year old son off at his friend's house he asked me: 'What are you going to do while I'm playing?' I answered: 'I'm going to yoga'. His response was: 'Good'."

- Audrey M., Colorado

***

"As an asthmatic child, I rarely took part in the normal activities that help develop physical skills, so I was never confident in my abilities. In adulthood, I went out of my way to avoid most sports; I was afraid to be embarrassed at not 'measuring up'.
One day, in my sixties, I saw a class for gentle yoga and I decided to give it a try. To my surprise I found out that I was actually good at it! As an unexpected bonus I found that yoga's breathing techniques have helped with my asthma.
After several years of yoga classes, I am confident about my body's strength and capability. Yoga has made it possible for me to challenge myself."

- Sue W., Colorado

"Yoga is really helping me to focus more on my strength and balance. I know the consistency is the key, and I have been working toward this goal. I love yoga classes. always feel calmer and more in tune with my body afterwards. It is important to me t have a good instructor in yoga class who is informative, supportive, and kind."

- Karen G., Colorad

***

"Since practicing yoga on a regular basis, my chiropractor and I have noticed a bi difference in my spine health, including better alignment and less back pain.
For most of my life I have measured 6'2", but in the past five years I had lo. approximately half an inch from my height, but after taking a couple of semesters o yoga, my last doctor's visit showed that I had regained the missing half an inch.

I have played tennis for 30+ years and I have improved my game considerably du to better flexibility and improved core strength, which I believe is due to regular yog practice"

- Mike L., Alask

I would like to thank all of my students that have attended my yoga classes, and truste me as a teacher on their yoga journey. Thank you for helping me to write this book My passion to endlessly explore yoga as a discipline and a way of life comes from your inspiration and commitment to yoga. Thank you for sharing your experience o yoga with me. Thank you for being a big part of my life.

Conclusion

"A journey of a thousand miles must begin with a single step"
- Lao Tzu

Practicing yoga is one of the ways to make profound changes in our lives that will have a ripple effect, and positively influence the lives of others. There is a lot of wisdom that we can learn from practicing yoga. It is a practice of self-discovery and self-exploration, as well as a practice of love, compassion, courage, and patience–qualities that the world needs right now. Lack of time, not enough resources, or too many obligations should not stand in the way of taking the first steps towards living better lives in a more harmonious world. The first step only takes a few minutes a day. Meaningful changes don't happen over night. They require taking one step at a time, one breath at a time, and in the practice of yoga–one pose at a time. If you are someone that has already taken the first step–keep going! This journey gets better and better as you take more and more steps. You can always change the direction of your path, or decide to move in a different direction as you approach a fork in the road. The most important thing is not to give up, and continue your commitment to your journey.

Our time is limited–whether we like it or not. This became a realization when my father passed away shortly before I finished writing this book. As I was saying good-bye to my Dad for the last time, I felt like a little girl. Even so, I knew that I must go on, and make use of the experiences, knowledge, and wisdom that I have learned since I was the little girl, to take the next steps, and persevere on my path.

I encourage you to join me on this journey–work with what you have, practice what you know, and learn what you can. Accomplish it all with love and gratitude for having another day and another opportunity to make a difference in your life, and in the lives of others.

Acknowledgments

I've been very fortunate to receive a lot of support from many people that have helped me throughout the journey of writing and publishing this book. I would have never been able to do it without you!

My husband–thank you for believing in me!

Regina Stribling, is very talented and dedicated editor, who has done a beautiful job revising this book, and sent me words of encouragement when I felt overwhelmed.

Kasia Hypsher, my friend, gifted graphic designer, and an amazing artist. Thank you for designing the book cover and book layout. Thank you for your patience and persistence in making my vision a reality.

Dr. Rhonda Cambridge-Phillip, MD, who supported me as my accountability partner, read the chapters as I finished each of them, made suggestions, and encouraged me to continue writing.

Family Garden, a non-profit Parenting Resource Center in Longmont, CO and its Founder and Executive Director, Debbie Lane, who made the yoga room available for my photography session.

Yoga postures models: Audrey, Liz, Courtney, Karen, Sheila, and my son Anthony. Thank you for making yourselves available, doing a great job presenting the poses, and sharing them with the readers of this book.

Dr. Nita Desai, a Board Certified Medical Doctor in Holistic Medicine, and a Certified Ayurvedic Practitioner, who was my first teacher that introduced me to the Ayurvedic wisdom and Eastern healing methods. For over 10 years Dr. Desai has helped my family and me with various health problems, inspired me with her knowledge and genuine care, gave me advice and hope, and always listened attentively.

My friends, teachers, and students from Fairbanks, Alaska, where I started my journey as a full time Yoga Instructor. Thank you for allowing me to learn from all of you bout how to become a passionate and thoughtful teacher. *Special Thanks* to: Gretchen Nolan, who was the owner of Infinite Yoga of Alaska, were I taught my first yoga lass; University of Alaska at Fairbanks, where I was proud to be a faculty member eaching yoga for three semesters; University of Alaska Yoga Club that gave me a hance to experience leading a yoga practice with more than 50 people of different ges, backgrounds, fitness levels, and beliefs.

Thank you to all my Students who have attended my yoga classes, workshops, and nini-retreats. I am grateful for each and every one of you. Every time I am ready to ead a class, I feel inspired by your wisdom, commitment, and kindness.

Resources

To help you become more comfortable with yoga poses and to continue enjoying th
benefits of your regular practice, I encourage you to look into the resources below. Th
resources will help you succeed in:

- finding a good yoga teacher in your area
- continuing to learning about yogic tools and practices continue learning abou
  yogic tools and practices
- experimenting with Ayurvedic cooking
- finding good quality Ayurvedic and other healthy products
- learning more about your constitution, choosing seasonal and local foods
- finding community that supports healthy living and provides a positiv
  environment

There are many resources that you will discover and research as you continue t
explore yoga. I have used the following resources for my personal and profession;
growth, as well as for writing this book. For a more complete list of references, pleas
check out the Reference List section in the back of this book.

Books

Yoga as Medicine – Timothy McCall, MD

Perfect Health for Kids – John Douillard

Yoga Body Diet – John Douillard

The 3-Season Diet – John Douillard

Yoga Wisdom & Practice – B.K.S. Iyengar

Relax and Renew: Restful Yoga for Stressful Times – Judith Hanson Lasater

The Heart of Yoga: Developing a Personal Practice – T.K.V. Desikachar

Perfect Health – Deepak Chopra

The Yoga of Breath: A Step-By-Step Guide to Pranayama – Richard Rosen

Cooking for Postpartum with Ayurveda – Heidi Nordlund

Eat Taste Heal: An Ayurvedic Guide and Cookbook for Modern Living – Thomas Yarema, MD, Daniel Rhoda, D.A.S, Chef Johnny Brannigan

Online Resources

www.yogajournal.com
Yoga Journal Magazine is the most popular yoga magazine. It offers a printed and an online version. It is a great source of information on yoga practice, health, wellness, and Ayurveda.

www.yogadirectory.com
An online database for yoga studios, retreats, healing services, publications, and other resources.

www.yogafinder.com
A website designed to help you find yoga classes, retreat centers, and events in specific geographical areas.

www.grokker.com
This website offers videos of many different styles of yoga as well as cooking demos.

www.chopra.com
Chopra Center, founded by Deepak Chopra MD, who is an Ayurvedic practitioner, author, public speaker and advocate for alternative medicine. Chopra Center offers an abundance of online information on healthy living including: blogs, programs, and webinars.

www.lifespa.com
Life Spa is founded by Dr. John Douillard, an Ayurvedic practitioner, author, and speaker. This site offers a wealth of information on yoga, fitness, Ayurveda, seasonal diets, and healthy living.

www.muditainstitute.com
Mudita Institute is an Australian based Ayurvedic training and education organization. The online site offers videos, courses, books, articles, and blogs.

www.yogauonline.com
Online yoga education for teachers and students offering videos, courses and blogs.

www.mercola.com
An alternative medicine website that provides many articles on health and wellness including the benefits of yoga and Ayurveda.

www.drweil.com
Dr. Weil is a pioneer in integrative medicine–a scientific approach similar to Ayurveda that includes the body, mind, and spirit in health and healing. Dr. Weil's website provides information on health prevention, healthy aging, herbs and supplements, health centers, cooking, exercise, meditation, and body and mind connection.

www.greenmedinfo.com
This website offers a large selection on health, alternative healing treatments, herbal remedies, nutrition, and body-mind therapies including yoga and Ayurveda.

www.hayhouse.com
This online site offers inspirational blogs, books, courses, apps, CDs, and events.

www.kriscarr.com
Kris Carr's website includes cleansing programs, healthy recipes, blogs and information on yoga, meditation, beauty, wellbeing, and personal success.

www.drmccall.com
Dr. McCall, the author of *Yoga as Medicine* offers many articles on yoga related topics, newsletters, and yoga therapy seminars.

www.mindbodygreen.com
This website offers information on yoga, meditation, fitness, nutrition, beauty, holistic health, and relationships.

nstitutes and Health Therapy Centers

Iimalayan Institute (himalayaninstitute.org) is located in Honesdale, PA. It is a holistic iealth center that offers many healing, educational and humanitarian programs. *Iimalayan Institute Botanicals* is a line of high quality Ayurvedic products.

Imega Institute for Holistic Studies (eomega.org) is located in Rhinebeck, NY. It iffers workshops, retreats, conferences, as well as online lectures, videos, and articles.

Kripalu Center for Yoga and Health (kripalu.org) is located in Stockbridge, MA. It iffers yoga teacher's trainings, on-site and online classes, healing arts' therapies, etreats, bodywork, and lifestyle consultations.

Chopra Center (chopra.com) was founded in 1996 by two physicians: Dr. Deepak Chopra and Dr. David Simon. Chopra Center is an Ayurvedic therapy center located in Carlsbad, CA. It offers many mind-body healing programs, Ayurvedic spa therapies, yoga, meditation, and medical consultations.

Life Spa (lifespa.com) is an Ayurvedic health spa located in Boulder, CO. It offers consultations with Dr. John Douillard, Ayurvedic therapies, herbs, supplements, and other Ayurvedic products.

East West Integrated Center (nitadesaimd.com) in Louisville, CO. Dr. Nita Desai is a physician and Ayurvedic Practitioner as well as the founder of the center. The center offers Ayurvedic consultations, Ayurvedic spa therapies, salt spa, Lymphatic Enhancement Therapy, and pain management.

Sanoviv (sanoviv.com) is located in Rosarito, Mexico on the Baja coast. It is a licensed hospital and health resort. Sanoviv offers many conventional, alternative, and integrative programs either to treat existing conditions or to improve and maintain wellness.

Hippocrates Health Institute (hippocratesinst.org) is located in West Palm Beach, FL. It offers educational and life transformational healing programs.

Integrative Restoration Institute (irest.us) offers worldwide trainings and retreats based on Yoga Nidra techniques. Their website has information on how to find an iRest trained teacher in specific geographical areas.

Shoshoni Yoga Retreat (shoshoni.org) is located in the Colorado Rockies. It offers yog teachers trainings, yoga and meditation workshops, retreats, and Ayurvedic therapie

Give Back Yoga Foundation (givebackyoga.org) is a non-profit yoga organization th offers programs and healing therapies for people with eating disorders, PTSD, cance as well as programs for veterans, prisoners, and specific trainings for yoga instructor

Ayurvedic foods and other healthy products

Pure Indian Foods (pureindianfoods.com) offers: spices, teas, ghee, oils (coconu black cumin, almond, sesame) grains, beans, and lentils.

Radiant Life (radiantlifecatalog.com) offers: coconut products, natural sweetener fats and oils, sprouted nuts and seeds, nut and seed butters, supplements, water filter personal and baby care products.

Mountain Rose Herbs (mountainroseherbs.com) offers: herbs, spices, teas, herb: extracts and tinctures, aromatherapy, home goods, hair and body care, elixirs an syrups.

Life Spa (lifespa.com) offers: herbs, supplements, Ayurvedic foods, test kits, bath an personal care, books, CDs, and DVDs.

Green Pasture (greenpasture.org) offers: coconut oil, coconut ghee, cod liver oil, butte oil, and skin care products.

Banyan Botanicals (banyanbotanicals.com) offers: Ayurvedic supplements, bul herbs, massage oils, soaps, syrups, sprays, liquid extracts, mung beans, ghee, Nasy oil, tongue scrapers, and neti pots.

Morrocco Method (mmhair.com) offers hair products: henna, shampoos, conditioner: brushes, elixirs, and body care products.

Yoga props

Gaiam (www.gaiam.com)

Hugger-Mugger (www.huggermugger.com)

Green Yoga (www.greenyoga.org)

Prana (www.prana.com)

Reference List

Chopra, Deepak. "5 Yoga Practices for Mind-Body Balance." *Chopra Center*.
http://www.chopra.com/ccl/5-yoga-practices-for-mind-body-balance.
Accessed 20 Jan. 2016.

"Digestive Diseases Statistics for the United States." *National Digestive Disease Information Clearinghouse,* National Institute of Diabetes and Digestive and Kidney Diseases,
https://www.niddk.nih.gov/health-information/health-statistics/Documents/Digestive_Disease_Stats_508.pdf. Accessed 30 Feb. 2016.

Doran, William J.D., "The Eight Limbs of Yoga, A Basic Overview."
Expressions of Spirit,
http://www.expressionsofspirit.com/yoga/eight-limbs.htm. Accessed 15 Mar. 2016

Douillard, John. *The Colorado Cleanse: 14 Day Ayurvedic Digestive Detox and Lymph Cleanse.* LifeSpa, 2016. E-book.
http://lifespa.com/wp-content/uploads/2012/11/short-home-cleanse_ebook_john-douillardslifespa_b.pdf.

Douillard, John. "Sleep Solutions for Your Body Type: Sleep Deeply, Wake Up Refreshed." LifeSpa, http://lifespa.com/sleep-solutions-for-your-body-type-sleep-deeply-wake-up-refreshed/. Accessed 1 Sept. 2016.

Douillard, John. "What Is Ayurveda? The Science, Body Types, LifeStyle and More." LifeSpa.
http://lifespa.com/about-lifespa/ayurveda/what-is-ayurveda/. Accessed 21 Mar. 2016

Edeslon, Mat."Take Two Carrots and Call Me in the Morning." *Hopkins Medicine Magazine. Winter 2010.*
http://www.hopkinsmedicine.org/hmn/w10/feature2.cfm. Accessed 9 Apr. 2016

Feng, Gia-Fu and English, Jane. *Lao Tsu - Tao Te Ching*, Wildwood House, 1991 Chapter 64.

Hall, Colin. "Hot and Bothered: The Hype, History, and Science of Hot Yoga." *Yoga International*,
https://yogainternational.com/article/view/hot-and-bothered-the-hype-history-and-science-of-hot-yoga. Accessed 21 Jan. 2016

Iyengar, B. K. S., Menuhin, Yehudi, and Patañjali. *Light on the Yoga Sutras of Patañjali.* Aquarian/Thorsons, 1993.

McCall, Timothy B. *Yoga as Medicine: The Yogic Prescription for Health & Healing: A Yoga Journal Book.* Bantam Dell, 2007.

MacGregor, Kino. "Ashtanga Yoga Guru Sri K. Pattabhi Jois, 1915-2009, In Memoriam" Ashtanga. http://www.ashtanga.com/html/macgregor3.html. Accessed 10 May 2016.

Mooventhan, A. and Nivethitha, L. "Scientific Evidence-Based Effects of Hydrotherapy on Various Systems of the Body." *North American Journal of Medical Sciences*, vol. 6, no. 5, 2014, pp.199-209.
http://www.najms.org/article.asp?issn=1947-2714;year=2014;volume=6;issue=5;spage=199;epage=209;aulast=Mooventhan. Accessed 18 Mar. 2016

Rosen, Richard, and Fraley, Kim. *The Yoga of Breath: A Step-by-step Guide to Pranayama*. Shambhala, 2002.

Ward, Becky. "14 Styles Of Yoga Explained Simply." *Mindbodygreen*,
http://www.mindbodygreen.com/0-8622/14-styles-of-yoga-explained-simply.html. Accessed 30 Aug. 2016.

Warner, Joe. "After Controversy in Houston, a Yoga Guru Resurrects His Practice in Denver." *Houston Press*. http://www.houstonpress.com/news/after-controversy-in-houston-a-yoga-guru-resurrects-his-practice-in-denver-6600444. Accessed 21 Jan. 2016.

Yarema, Thomas, Rhoda, Daniel, Brannigan, Johnny, and Ouellette, Ed. *Eat-taste-heal: An Ayurvedic Guidebook and Cookbook for Modern Living.*
Five Elements, 2006.

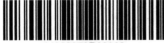

61858878R00062

Made in the USA
Charleston, SC
28 September 2016